PHYSICAL
EXAMINATION
OF
THE JOINTS

WILLIAM P. BEETHAM, Jr., M.D., A.A.C.P.

Former Fellow in Medicine,
Mayo Graduate School of Medicine,
University of Minnesota

HOWARD F. POLLEY, M.D., M.S. in Medicine, F.A.C.P.

Head of a Section of Medicine
(Rheumatic Diseases), Mayo Clinic;
Professor of Medicine,
Mayo Graduate School of Medicine,
University of Minnesota

CHARLES H. SLOCUMB, M.D., M.S. in Pathology

Senior Consultant in a Section of Medicine
(Rheumatic Diseases), Mayo Clinic;
Professor of Medicine,
Mayo Graduate School of Medicine,
University of Minnesota

WALT F. WEAVER, M.D., M.S. in Medicine, A.A.C.P.

Former Fellow in Medicine,
Mayo Graduate School of Medicine,
University of Minnesota

Rochester, Minnesota

With 15 Anatomic Drawings by RUSSELL L. DRAKE,
Emeritus Director of Mayo Clinic Section of Medical Illustrations

PHYSICAL
EXAMINATION
OF
THE JOINTS

W. B. SAUNDERS COMPANY
PHILADELPHIA AND LONDON,

W. B. Saunders Company: West Washington Square
                          Philadelphia, Pa. 19105

                          12 Dyott Street
                          London, W.C.1

Reprinted October, 1965 and May, 1966

Physical Examination of the Joints

"Was man weiss man sieht."

What one knows one sees.

Goethe

PREFACE

THIS MONOGRAPH is intended for physicians and students who wish an elementary, comprehensive guide for conducting the physical examination of joints and for evaluating involvement of the joints in the various rheumatic diseases.

The technics of examination are described in detail, as the ability to perform the joint examination accurately is helpful and in most instances even essential for establishing the correct diagnosis. In discussion of the technic of examining joints only the pertinent anatomic features are presented. The anatomy of the synovial membrane is described in detail because it is of particular importance in the examination of the patient with an involved joint and because it is often poorly understood. Many nonarticular physical signs present in rheumatic diseases are essentially part of general physical diagnosis; these are not described herein. Likewise the details of the history of the patient with rheumatic disease, important as they are in the evaluation and treatment of the patient, are beyond the scope of this undertaking.

The available medical literature has been correlated with the experiences and concepts of the authors and other consultants in rheumatology at the Mayo Clinic. At the end of each section describing the examination of a particular joint or a group of related joints, a list of references is supplied for those who may desire additional information.

The material in this text is arranged according to objective signs rather than disease entities. It is concerned primarily with recognition and localization of disease and only secondarily with the diagnostic classification of the disease processes. There is intentional repetition in the text for the purpose of relating anatomy to inspection as well as to palpation in the physical examination of the various joints and to minimize the need of cross reference as a convenience for the reader.

This monograph is the result of many persons' efforts. We are particularly indebted to Mr. Russell L. Drake and Mr. John M. Hutcheson, artists at the Mayo Clinic and the Mayo Foundation, for their contributions. Drawings of the joints, bursae, and synovial mem-

branes were done by Mr. Drake and Mr. Hutcheson and the line drawings and range of motion charts were done by Mr. Hutcheson. We
also wish to thank the Section of Photography for their help in obtaining
many of the photographs. Miss M. Katharine Smith from the Section
of Publications graciously and skillfully edited the manuscript.

WILLIAM P. BEETHAM, JR.
HOWARD F. POLLEY
CHARLES H. SLOCUMB
WALT F. WEAVER

CONTENTS

CONTENTS

CHAPTER ONE

INTRODUCTION TO EXAMINATION OF THE JOINTS

AMERICAN RHEUMATISM ASSOCIATION'S NOMENCLA-
TURE AND CLASSIFICATION OF ARTHRITIS AND
RHEUMATISM (TENTATIVE)

EXAMINATION OF THE JOINTS

> Structure and Classification of Joints
> > *Plane joints*
> > *Spheroidal joints*
> > *Cotylic joints*
> > *Hinge joints*
> > *Condylar joints*
> > *Trochoid or pivot joints*
> > *Sellar joints*
> Systematic Method of Examination
> Important Physical Signs of Arthritis
> > *Swelling*
> > *Tenderness*
> > *Range of motion*
> > *Other important physical signs*

THE JOINT CHART

> Purpose and Essential Features
> Method
> > *Abbreviations*
> Interpretation of Chart (Table 1)
> An Abbreviated Record

The ability to recognize what can be seen is a rewarding diagnostic dividend. Since the joints and other musculoskeletal structures are derived from the mesenchyme, which is characterized by a potential for marked cellular reactivity in the presence of disease, and since many of these are near the surface of the body, the observing examiner is provided an excellent opportunity for obtaining significant information about many diseases.

1

To help detect and localize disease within or outside of the joint, the technics of physical examination of the joints and related structures will be correlated with articular anatomy throughout this monograph. The details of such examination are particularly helpful in analyzing the symptoms and signs of the rheumatic component of diseases which are localized to an articular area or to the musculoskeletal system or may be an expression of generalized or systemic diseases.

Accurate diagnosis as well as adequate care of the patient with articular disease also requires complete general medical examination in addition to thorough study of the joints and adjacent tissues. The value of careful physical examination of the joints and related musculo-skeletal structures is indicated by the broad spectrum of diseases and conditions that symptomatically and objectively affect joints; this is illustrated by the variety of diseases included in a tentative nomenclature and classification of arthritis and rheumatism proposed recently (1963) by the American Rheumatism Association that follows. Knowledge of the conditions in this list can aid the examining physician in considering the diagnostic possibilities in individual patients.

AMERICAN RHEUMATISM ASSOCIATION'S NOMENCLATURE AND CLASSIFICATION OF ARTHRITIS AND RHEUMATISM (TENTATIVE)*

  I. Polyarthritis of unknown etiology
    A. Rheumatoid arthritis
    B. Juvenile rheumatoid arthritis (Still's disease)
    C. Ankylosing spondylitis
    D. Psoriatic arthritis
    E. Reiter's syndrome
    F. Others
 II. "Connective tissue" disorders
    A. Systemic lupus erythematosus
    B. Periarteritis nodosa
    C. Scleroderma (progressive systemic sclerosis)
    D. Polymyositis and dermatomyositis
    E. Others
III. Rheumatic fever
 IV. Degenerative joint disease (osteoarthritis, osteoarthrosis)
    A. Primary
    B. Secondary
  V. Non-articular rheumatism
    A. Fibrositis
    B. Intervertebral disc and low back syndromes
    C. Myositis and myalgia
    D. Tendinitis and peritendinitis (bursitis)
    E. Tenosynovitis
    F. Fasciitis

---

* Reprinted from Bulletin of Rheumatic Disease 14:339–340 (Mar.) 1964.

  G. Carpal tunnel syndrome
  H. Others
   (See also shoulder-hand syndrome, VIII E)
 VI. Diseases with which arthritis is frequently associated
  A. Sarcoidosis
  B. Relapsing polychondritis
  C. Henoch-Schönlein syndrome
  D. Ulcerative colitis
  E. Regional ileitis
  F. Whipple's disease
  G. Sjögren's syndrome
  H. Familial Mediterranean fever
  I. Others
   (See also psoriatic arthritis, I D)
 VII. [Arthritis] associated with known infectious agents
  A. Bacterial
   1. Brucella
   2. Gonococcus
   3. Mycobacterium tuberculosis
   4. Pneumococcus
   5. Salmonella
   6. Staphylococcus
   7. Streptobacillus moniliformis (Haverhill fever)
   8. Treponema pallidum (syphilis)
   9. Treponema pertenue (yaws)
   10. Others
  B. Rickettsial
  C. Viral
  D. Fungal
  E. Parasitic
   (See also rheumatic fever, III)
 VIII. Traumatic and/or neurogenic disorders
  A. Traumatic arthritis (viz., the result of direct trauma)
  B. Lues (tertiary syphilis)
  C. Diabetes
  D. Syringomyelia
  E. Shoulder-hand syndrome
  F. Mechanical derangements of joints
  G. Others
   (See also degenerative joint disease; IV; carpal tunnel, syndrome V G)
 IX. [Disease] associated with known biochemical or endocrine abnormalities
  A. Gout
  B. Ochronosis
  C. Hemophilia
  D. Hemoglobinopathy (e.g., sickle cell disease)
  E. Agammaglobulinemia
  F. Gaucher's disease
  G. Hyperparathyroidism
  H. Acromegaly
  I. Hypothyroidism
  J. Scurvy (hypovitaminosis C)
  K. Xanthoma tuberosum
  L. Others
   (See also multiple myeloma, X G; Hurler's syndrome, XII C)

X. Tumor and tumor-like conditions
    A. Synovioma
    B. Pigmented villonodular synovitis
    C. Giant cell tumor of tendon sheath
    D. Primary juxta-articular bone tumors
    E. Metastatic [tumors]
    F. Leukemia
    G. Multiple myeloma
    H. Benign tumors of articular tissue
    I. Others
      (See also hypertrophic osteoarthropathy, XIII G)
XI. Allergy and drug reactions
    A. Arthritis due to specific allergens (e.g., serum sickness)
    B. Arthritis due to drugs (e.g., hydralazine syndrome)
    C. Others
XII. Inherited and congenital disorders
    A. Marfan's syndrome
    B. Ehlers-Danlos syndrome
    C. Hurler's syndrome
    D. Congenital hip dysplasia
    E. Morquio's disease
    F. Others
XIII. Miscellaneous disorders
    A. Amyloidosis
    B. Aseptic necrosis of bone
    C. Behcet's syndrome
    D. Chondrocalcinosis (pseudo-gout)
    E. Erythema multiforme (Stevens-Johnson syndrome)
    F. Erythema nodosum
    G. Hypertrophic osteoarthropathy
    H. Juvenile osteochondritis
    I. Osteochondritis dissecans
    J. Reticulohistiocytosis of joints (lipoid dermato-arthritis)
    K. Tietze's disease
    L. Others

EXAMINATION OF THE JOINTS

The physical examination of the arthritic patient actually begins when the physician first sees the patient and obtains useful information from the general appearance and attitudes of the patient, gross deformities, state of nutrition, gait, and body position. For example, observations can be made of the patient's ability to get out of a chair or bed, to climb up or down stairs, to care for himself, and to perform the usual daily functions such as feeding, writing, and dressing. Information regarding function of muscles and joints is obtained from, and should be included in, the inquiry into the patient's history.

In the clinical evaluation of joints the variations among individuals without definite articular abnormalities are of interest and should be considered. The only really reliable method of learning how to

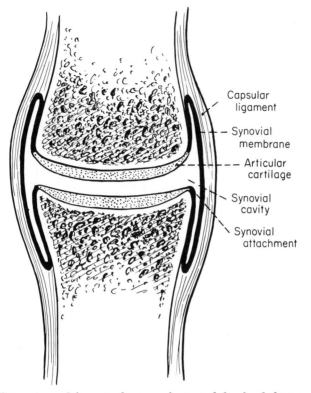

Figure 1.   Schematic diagram of a typical diarthrodial joint.

examine joints and remaining familiar with the variations of normality is by repeated experience. The examiner must be aware of the variations produced by age, sex, body habitus, and occupation as well as those resulting from heredity and disease.

Structure and Classification of Joints

Interpretation of the examination of the joints is facilitated by an understanding of the significant anatomic aspects of the joints of the body. Joints or articulations are formed wherever bones of the skeleton are joined to one another.

Joints are of three main types: (1) synarthroses (immovable articulations), (2) amphiarthroses (slightly movable articulations), and (3) diarthroses (freely movable articulations). In synarthrotic joints the bones are joined and held together by fibrous tissue or cartilage. The surfaces of the joined bones are in almost direct contact with each other and this close contact allows no appreciable motion. The joints between the bones of the skull are examples of synarthroses. The bony surfaces of amphiarthrotic joints are united by fibrocartilaginous disks, as in the articulations between vertebral bodies, or are joined by a fibrous interosseous ligament, as in the inferior tibiofibular articulation. Diarthroses are freely movable, synovial-lined joints in which the bones are separated from each other by a fluid-containing cavity. The knee joint is an example. Diarthrodial joints are the most common joints in the body and are the joints with which the rheumatologist is particularly concerned. In this and subsequent chapters the term "joint" will refer to a diarthrodial joint, unless otherwise stated.

The articulating ends of the bones forming a diarthrodial joint are covered by cartilage and are enclosed in a capsule of fibrous tissue. The joint capsule is strengthened by strong ligaments extending between the bones of the joint. The articular cartilage, which normally is resilient, acts as a cushion between the bones, and the smooth surface of the cartilage allows ease of movement. The synovial membrane lines the inner surface of the fibrous capsule, forms the inner lining of the joint, and is attached at the margins of the articular cartilages. The synovial membrane between these margins is composed of folds and pouches which facilitate or allow movement of the joint (Fig. 1). Normally only a small amount of synovial fluid is present within the confines of the synovial membrane to provide lubrication of the inner surface of the joint. The volume of synovial fluid varies somewhat from joint to joint, but even in the largest peripheral joint, the knee, the recoverable volume normally can vary from none, in cases in which no free fluid can be aspirated although the surfaces of the joint are moist from a thin layer of viscous fluid, to about 3.5 ml. of free fluid.

Diarthrodial or synovial joints have been classified further according to the shapes of the surfaces that articulate. The shape of the articulating surface, in turn, determines the type and extent of motion in the joint. According to Barnett and associates[1] there are seven types or forms of articulating surfaces: plane, spheroidal, cotylic, hinge, condylar, trochoid, and sellar. This descriptive classification was adopted and recommended for general use by the VIth International Congress of Anatomists in Paris in 1955.

Plane Joints. Plane joints allow only gliding movements. Gliding movement is the simplest type of joint movement that can take place and consists of one surface moving over another without any rotatory or angular movement. Articular surfaces of this type of joint are supposed to be plane or flat. Actually they are often slightly curved. The slight movement in this type of joint is limited by the ligaments and bony processes surrounding the articulation. The carpal joints (except those of the capitate with the navicular and the lunate) and the tarsal joints (except that between the talus and navicular) are examples of this type of diarthrodial joint.

Spheroidal Joints. Spheroidal joints also are called ball-and-socket joints since they are formed by the articulation of a rounded convex surface with a cuplike cavity. The distal bone of the joint is capable of a wide variety of movements including flexion, extension, abduction, adduction, rotation, and circumduction. The shoulder and hip joints are familiar examples of this form of articulation.

Cotylic Joints. These joints are similar to spheroidal joints, but the articular surfaces resemble an ellipse rather than a circle. Cotylic joints, therefore, are referred to also as ellipsoid joints and are more restricted in motion than spheroidal joints since they permit flexion, extension, abduction, adduction, and circumflexion, but not axial rotation. The convex surface in a cotylic joint is somewhat longer in one direction and relatively shorter in the direction perpendicular to the long one, producing an ovoid articular surface which is received into an elliptical cavity that forms the concave surface of the joint. Cotylic joints are further subdivided according to whether they are simple or compound. A *simple cotylic joint* is one whose articular capsule encloses only one pair of articulating surfaces while in a *compound cotylic joint* the articular capsule encloses more than one pair of articulating surfaces. The metacarpophalangeal joints of the hand are examples of simple cotylic joints, and the radiocarpal (wrist) joint is an example of a compound cotylic joint.

Hinge Joints. These joints permit motion in only one plane, flexion and extension. A hinge joint is described also as "ginglymus." The articular surfaces of this type of joint are joined together by strong collateral ligaments which restrict lateral movement, but the extent of flexion and extension in the joint may be considerable. The best examples of hinge joints are the interphalangeal joints of the hand and foot and the humero-ulnar (elbow) joint. In these joints the range of flexion exceeds that of extension, but extension is considered to occur when the flexed joint is returned to its resting position.

Condylar Joints. In condylar joints one bone articulates with the other by two distinct articular surfaces whose movements are not dissociable. Each of these articular surfaces is referred to as a condyle. Either the convex or concave surface of the joint may be termed a "condyle"; thus the knee has tibial condyles as well as femoral condyles. Condylar joints resemble hinge joints in their movements but differ from them in the structure of their articular surfaces. The articular condyles of this type of joint may be close together and enclosed in the same articular capsule, as in the knee joint, or they may be widely separated and enclosed in separate articular capsules, as in the paired temporomandibular joints.

Trochoid or Pivot Joints. In trochoid or pivot joints the movement of the joint is limited to rotation. This type of joint is formed by a bony pivotlike process turning within a ring or a ring turning around a bony pivot. The ring portion of the joint is formed partly by bone and partly by a fibrous ligament. The proximal radio-ulnar joint is

7

a trochoid joint in which the radial head rotates within the ring formed by the radial notch of the ulna and the annular ligament. The atlanto-odontal joint (medial atlanto-axial joint) is an example of a trochoid joint in which the ring, formed by the anterior arch and transverse ligament of the atlas, rotates around the odontoid process of the axis.

Sellar Joints. These have saddle-shaped articular surfaces. In this form of joint, a convex surface articulates with a concave surface in such a manner as to allow flexion, extension, abduction, adduction, and circumduction, but no axial rotation. The classic example of a sellar joint is the carpometacarpal joint of the thumb.

Systematic Method of Examination

A systematic method of examining joints is the quickest and easiest way of obtaining the available information. The examiner often begins with the joints of the upper extremity and proceeds to the joints of the trunk and the lower extremity, but a reverse of this procedure is just as effective and is preferred on some occasions. In either instance corresponding joints are compared systematically with each other and with respect to normalcy or abnormality for the particular joint. Inspection and palpation supplement each other; they usually can be performed together and can be followed by evaluation of joint motion.

The patient should be as comfortable as possible. Since muscles and tendons overlie and surround most joints, they must be as soft and relaxed as possible if the physician is to examine the underlying joint adequately. Rough or forceful handling of inflamed joints may cause not only severe pain but also muscle spasm and loss of patient cooperation so that further examination becomes difficult or unreliable. Excessive muscle spasm and guarding can usually be avoided by firm support of the area being examined and gentle handling of painful joint areas. When the examination of a painful joint requires moving it from the neutral and relaxed position, care should be taken to return the extremity slowly to a comfortable position before withdrawing the examiner's support; quick motions should be avoided. A simple explanation to the patient of what is being done or is to be done during the examination is reassuring and often is necessary to obtain reliable observations.

Important Physical Signs of Arthritis

"Arthritis" is a general term used to describe the existence of disease *within* the joint itself. Since a typical diarthrodial joint consists of subchondral bone, articular cartilage, and a synovial membrane, one

8

or more of these structures must be affected to permit accurate use of the term "arthritis." Synovitis or inflammation of the synovial membrane, from whatever cause, is therefore synonymous with arthritis, although arthritis by definition may also include involvement of the articular cartilage or subchondral bone or both with or without synovitis. However, the presence or absence of synovitis is often the most accessible and therefore the most important physical finding in the detection of arthritis. Either thickening of the synovial membrane or articular effusion is indicative of synovitis, and often both are present simultaneously in the same joint. The most common signs of articular synovitis are swelling, tenderness, and limitation of motion.

Swelling. Swelling about a joint may be caused by intra-articular effusion, synovial thickening, periarticular soft-tissue inflammation such as bursitis or tendinitis, bony enlargement, or extra-articular fat pads. These conditions need to be differentiated from one another. Soft-tissue swelling may be either intra-articular or extra-articular in origin. It is particularly important to differentiate intra-articular soft-tissue swelling from extra-articular or periarticular involvement since intra-articular soft-tissue swelling is indicative of arthritis (synovitis). The term "joint enlargement" is a generalization which should be avoided as it does not distinguish joint swelling, periarticular swelling, and bony enlargement. Although muscle atrophy makes synovial effusion relatively more evident, it also may give a misleading impression of bony enlargement of a joint.

The synovial membrane is the "soft tissue" of the joint and is commonly inflamed, infected, irritated, or otherwise involved early in various arthritic processes. The resulting change in the synovial membrane may be detected by careful physical examination earlier than the involvement of other affected, hard, articular structures. Although synovial thickening and effusion are frequently associated, the examiner should try to recognize the extent of each even though this is not always possible.

Familiarity with the anatomic configuration of the synovial membrane in various joints aids in differentiating the soft-tissue swelling due to synovitis (articular effusion or synovial thickening) from the swelling of periarticular tissues. On physical examination the presence of an effusion of a joint ("joint fluid") is often demonstrated by a visible or a palpable bulging of the joint capsule or by both. Since the synovial fluid lies in a closed sac, compression of one portion of this sac causes the fluid to shift within the sac and adds to the distention of the sac elsewhere. A thickened synovial membrane with or without palpable effusion indicates arthritis (synovitis), and fluid in the joint also indicates arthritis (synovitis) even though the synovial membrane may not be palpably thickened. The normal synovial membrane is not palpable, whereas the thickened or abnormal synovial membrane

9

may have a "doughy" or "boggy" consistency on palpation. In some joints the margin of the synovial membrane can be delineated on physical examination by compressing synovial fluid into one of the extreme limits of its reflection. The edge of the resulting bulge thus may be palpated more easily and represents a summation of the synovial membrane and the movable fluid within the synovial cavity. If this palpable edge is within the anatomic confines of the synovial membrane and disappears on release of the compression, the distention may be regarded as representing synovial effusion; if it persists, it is indicative of a thickened synovial membrane. However, reliable differentiation between synovial thickening and effusion is not always possible by physical examination. There is a small amount of synovial fluid present in a normal joint, but it is not palpable; palpable fluid in a joint is abnormal and indicates synovitis.

The examiner should be able to determine by palpation and inspection whether or not a patient has joint swelling. Although it is at times difficult to make a decision from physical examination, there is no in-between state. The presence of swelling is a definite and significant finding; therefore, terms such as "questionable swelling" and "possible swelling" used to conceal uncertainty should be avoided. Repetition of the examination and experience with accurate examination of joints will aid in the determination of whether synovitis is present or not.

Tenderness. Localization of tenderness by palpation should make it apparent whether the reaction is intra-articular or in periarticular structures such as fat pads, tendon attachments, ligaments, bursae, muscles, or skin. Because tenderness is at least partly a subjective reaction, the degree of tenderness should be correlated with the emotional state of the patient. Proper interpretation of the presence of tenderness on palpation requires adequate relaxation of the muscles and tendons in the area being examined. Excessive muscle spasm may make reliable evaluation of tenderness difficult or impossible.

When possible, the examiner should try to differentiate between the pain due to distention of the synovial membrane and the pain caused by a localized inflammatory process in soft tissues. This can usually be done during the physical examination by careful localization of tender areas to specific anatomic structures. Recognition of the localization of inflammatory processes in either the synovial membrane or the perisynovial tissues or both is important because in the course of certain rheumatic diseases such as episodic rheumatoid arthritis, gout, acute rheumatic fever, palindromic rheumatism, and lupus erythematosus, inflammatory perisynovial or extra-articular reactions may be more significant or may be an earlier finding than synovial distention.

Range of Motion. The range as well as the type of motion in a normal joint depends on the shape of the articular surfaces (as

10

described earlier in this chapter), the restraining effect of supporting ligaments, and the control exerted by muscles acting on the joint. Since limitation of motion may be a common manifestation of articular disease, it is important to know the normal type and range of motion in order to detect limitation of motion due to abnormalities of the joint or adjacent structures. In subsequent chapters, the type and range of motion normally present in each joint are described, but generally the emphasis in the text will be on limitation of motion because of its importance and significance as a physical finding on examination of joints.

Limitation of motion may occur on either active or passive motion. In the former instance, motion is restricted when the patient attempts voluntary movement of a part; in the latter, motion is restricted when the examiner attempts movement of a part with the patient's muscles relaxed. When the active and passive ranges of motion are not equal, the passive range is usually greater and is thus the more reliable indication of the actual range of motion. However, the active range of motion should be observed before the passive range of motion is determined whenever possible. To some extent information with regard to active range of motion becomes evident from the history, including a detailed description of the activities of daily living. This information is supplemented by observations made during physical examination. Discrepancies between active and passive ranges of motion may give valuable clues to abnormalities of the joints. A patient may restrict the range of passive motion if he fears that the examiner may hurt him and thus may have a greater range of active motion. On the other hand, he may not be able to move a joint fully because of pain from one or another of the tissues used mechanically to produce specific motions (for example, from swollen bursa, nodular tendon sheaths, torn or ruptured tendons, or otherwise affected tendons, tendon sheaths, or tendinous attachments) or because of muscle weakness or misuse of antagonist muscles. Yet with careful examination in these instances the range of passive motion may be nearly normal. Normally the ranges of active and of passive motion should be approximately the same if only intraarticular disease is present.

Limitation of joint motion may be transient or permanent. Transient (reversible) limitation of motion may be due to (1) muscle spasm from fear or pain, (2) periarticular, fibrositic gelling which improves with repeated movements, (3) intra-articular effusion and synovitis, (4) "locking" secondary to loose bodies in a joint, defects or disorders of the meniscus, or malposition of tendons, and (5) fibrous proliferation producing intra-articular or periarticular adhesions, tenosynovitis, or contractures of muscle, fascia, and tendons. Permanent limitation of motion may be due to intra-articular or extra-articular causes. The former include fibrous or bony ankylosis, destruction of articular surfaces, subluxation, or impingement of bony spurs. Extra-

11

articular causes may be tightening of the articular capsule or tendinous and fascial contractures.

Other Important Physical Signs. These include temperature and color changes in the skin over a joint, crepitation, and deformity. *Changes in temperature and color* can best be interpreted by comparison with the opposite joint. Increase in warmth and redness of the skin is a variable finding which may or may not be apparent in the presence of articular synovitis.

Crepitation is a palpable or audible grating or crunching sensation produced by motion. It may or may not be accompanied by discomfort. Crepitation occurs when roughened articular or extra-articular surfaces are rubbed together either by active motion or by manual compression in the course of examination. Crepitation from within the joint should be differentiated from cracking sounds due to the slipping of ligaments or tendons over bony surfaces during motion.

Deformity may occur as bony enlargement, articular subluxation, contracture, and ankylosis in abnormal positions.

The application and interpretation of these physical signs as they relate more specifically to the various joints will be described in later chapters.

THE JOINT CHART

Purpose and Essential Features

A permanent record of examinations of the joints is of particular help in determining progress of arthritic disease. A satisfactory chart for recording observations made during examination of the joints and also for prompting the examiner to make a complete record (1) provides the necessary completeness, (2) is convenient, and (3) is adaptable for use by different examiners. It contains space for a complete description of swelling, tenderness, and limitation of motion of each joint whether normal or abnormal and for other important articular or periarticular findings. Such a chart is especially useful for the systematic recording of information obtained in research or investigative studies of patients whose long-term course must be followed closely. A more abbreviated chart indicating and recording only abnormal findings may be satisfactory for other requirements. A generally satisfactory detailed chart is illustrated in Table 1. A shorter method of recording these data will be described also.

Method

Abbreviations. To avoid a cumbersome chart, abbreviations are necessary. Abbreviations for the names of joints that are used in the chart are as follows: temporomandibular (T-M), sternoclavicular

Table 1. *Example of Chart for Recording Joint Examination**

Name_____Date_____

Joint	Right (Rt.)				Left (Lt.)			
	S	T	L	Comments	S	T	L	Comments
T-M	0	0	0		0	0	0	
S-C	0	0	0		0	0	0	
A-C	0	0	0		0	0	0	
Sh	0	2		Abd. 60° (or grade 1+)	0	0	0	
				Ext. rot. 60° (or grade 1+)				
				Int. rot. 60° (or grade 1+)				
Elb	0	0	0		0	0	0	
Wr	1+	1−		Dorsiflexion 35° (or grade 2)	0	0	0	
MCP	0	0	0 ⎫	MCP$_2$	1	1−	0 ⎫	
PIP	0	0	0 ⎬ Fist 100%	PIP$_2$	1+	0	0 ⎬ Fist 100%	
DIP	0	0	0 ⎭		0	0	0 ⎭	
Hip	0	0	0		0	0	0	
Kn	1	1		Ext. 15° (or grade 1)	0	0	0	
				Flex. 115° (or grade 1)				
Ank	0	0	0		0	0	0	
S-T	0	0	0		0	0	0	
MTP	0	0	0	MTP$_2$	1	1	0	
PIP	0	0	0		0	0	0	
DIP	0	0	0		0	0	0	
Spine								

Cervical

    Atlas (vertebrae 1 & 2)   T$_0$ L$_0$

    Vertebrae 3-7   T$_0$ L$_0$

Thoracic

    Costochondral   T$_0$ L$_0$

    Chest expansion   12.5 cm. (5 in.)

Lumbar   T$_0$ L$_0$

    Lumbosacral   T$_0$ L$_0$

Sacro-iliac   T$_0$

Coccyx   T$_0$

Posture__Mild upper thoracic rounding

Gait__Normal

                    Examiner_____

* For explanation of abbreviations, see text.

(S-C), costochondral (C-C), acromioclavicular (A-C), shoulder (Sh), elbow (Elb), wrist (Wr), metacarpophalangeal (MCP), proximal interphalangeal (PIP), distal interphalangeal (DIP), sacro-iliac (S-I), hip (no abbreviation necessary), knee (Kn), ankle (Ank), subtalar (S-T), and metatarsophalangeal (MTP), respectively. Other appropriate abbreviations may be used if desired. The digits are numbered 1 through 5 starting with the thumb in the case of the hand and with the great toe of the foot. Some orthopedic surgeons prefer to designate individual fingers by description rather than by the numbering of 1 through 5 as follows: thumb, index finger, middle finger, ring finger and little finger.

13

In recording the degree of swelling (S), tenderness (T), and limitation of motion (L) of a joint, a quantitative estimate of gradation based on a system of grades from 0 to 4 is convenient and may be used as follows: 0 means normal; 1, mildly abnormal; 2, moderately abnormal; 3, markedly abnormal; and 4, maximally abnormal. This grading is used in Table 1.

The abbreviation, S, as used in the chart refers to synovial swelling, thickening or effusion, or combinations thereof. If extra-articular edema or capsular, bursal, or osseous enlargement is present, a specific description of this is needed to avoid confusion in the use of the abbreviation, S, as the indicator for synovial swelling. Synovial swelling is best evaluated by the simultaneous use of both inspection and palpation. Swelling of grade 1 severity, designated in the chart in Table 1, as "1" in the column "S" and conveniently referred to as "S_1," may not be apparent on casual inspection but should be recognizable to an experienced examiner. Swelling of grades 2, 3, and 4 severity (S_2, S_3, and S_4, respectively) indicates increasing degrees of visible distention or thickening of the synovial membrane. Swelling of grade 1 or 2 is much more frequently observed than swelling of grade 3 or 4; swelling of grade 4 is actually rare. Because swelling of grade 1 or 2 occurs frequently, some examiners prefer to use divisions within these grades, such as 1—, 1+, 2— and 2+, conveniently referred to as S_{1-}, S_{1+}, S_{2-}, and S_{2+}, to indicate variations which can be observed, rather than to use grades 3 and 4 when these extremes of swelling are not precisely justified. Since the synovial membrane (and articular capsule) is generally less capable of marked distention when swelling occurs acutely than when swelling develops chronically, the extreme degrees of synovial swelling are more often found when the synovitis has developed slowly or been present chronically. In individual instances the degree of swelling may be the same as, or disproportionately greater or lesser than, the amount of tenderness. The grade of swelling and the grade of tenderness (see below) are coexisting indicators of articular abnormalities but need to be evaluated separately.

T generally refers to tenderness of the synovial membranes or perisynovial capsule or to both. Tenderness of other structures needs to be specifically differentiated and designated accordingly (for example, tendons, fat pads, and semilunar cartilages). Tenderness of grade 1 severity (T_1) indicates slight or mild tolerable discomfort on palpation. Grade 2 tenderness (T_2) indicates more severe pain on ordinary palpation which the patient prefers not to tolerate. Grade 3 tenderness (T_3) describes marked and even more intolerable pain with even light palpation or pressure. Grade 4 tenderness (T_4) is less commonly encountered and indicates pain which may be caused by a mild stimulus such as blowing air onto the joint, light touch, slight motion of the skin overlying the joint, or the vibration of heavy footsteps nearby. It should

14

be noted also whether pain is present during rest or only with movement. Some observers use + and − to denote slight variations within a grade when describing the severity of tenderness in a joint. For example, tenderness, grade 2 (T_2), may be used to indicate pain on palpation which the patient prefers not to tolerate but from which he does not pull away involuntarily, whereas T_{2+} is indicative of pain from which the patient involuntarily withdraws the examined joint, but the pain is still less than that graded 3.

In the case of *limitation of motion* (L), grade 1 may be used to indicate about 25 per cent loss of motion; grade 2, about 50 per cent; grade 3, about 75 per cent; and grade 4, 100 per cent or complete ankylosis. Again the symbols + and − may be used to denote variations within a grade; thus a 35 per cent loss of motion would equal grade 1+ and an 85 per cent loss of motion would equal grade 3+. The range of motion of the joints in degrees may be recorded in addition to, or in preference to, grading by the numerical scale and is a more accurate recording of the motion. In order to maintain consistency and simplicity in measuring the range of joint motion, the neutral position of a joint has been designated as "0 degrees" ("0°" in chart) throughout the text, even though some physicians prefer to designate the neutral position as "180 degrees" in certain joints (for example, the knee and the elbow). Generally, motion in the knee, finger joints, and elbow is suited to recording by measurement in degrees whereas motion in the wrist, ankle, metatarsophalangeal joints, and temporomandibular joints can be graded more conveniently and just as satisfactorily. In the shoulder and hip, abduction and adduction are often best measured in degrees, but rotation is measured either by degrees or by gradations.

Interpretation of the Chart (Table 1)

The chart illustrated in Table 1 shows the presence of a moderately tender and limited right shoulder; a mildly swollen (synovial) and tender right wrist with moderate limitation of dorsiflexion; a slightly swollen (synovial) and tender metacarpophalangeal joint of the left second finger; a mildly swollen (synovial) proximal interphalangeal joint of the left second finger; a slightly swollen (synovial) and tender right knee with slight limitation of motion in both extension and flexion; and a mildly swollen (synovial) and tender metatarsophalangeal joint of the left second toe.

As mentioned earlier, comments describing swelling or tenderness are often necessary in addition to grading for greater specificity. Thus tenderness in the shoulder might be due to involvement of the subdeltoid portion of the subacromial bursa, the bicipital extension (or out-pouching) of the articular synovial membrane, the rotator cuff of the shoulder, or the synovial membrane of the glenohumeral joint, and the specific site would need to be noted. An additional statement to interpret and record observations relative to muscular weakness, cutaneous or subcutaneous contractures, nodules, local heat and color changes, bursal or tenosynovial swelling, and tenderness of fibrous attachments should be made when any of these conditions is present.

An Abbreviated Record

If a more abbreviated record were being used, the joint examination given in detail in Table 1 could be recorded simply and briefly as Rt. Sh S_0, T_2, L_{1+}; Rt. Wr S_{1+}, T_{1-}, L_2; Lt. MCP_2, S_1, T_{1-}, L_0; Lt. PIP_2, S_{1+}, T_0, L_0; Rt. Kn, S_1, T_1, L_1 (lacks 15° of extension); Lt. MTP_2 S_1, T_1, L_0. The omission of certain detailed and important data is avoided by use of the more detailed information when indicated. For other useful methods of recording the joint examination, reference may be made to the following sources:

1. Lansbury, John: Methods for Evaluating Rheumatoid Arthritis. In Hollander, J. L.: Arthritis and Allied Conditions: A Textbook of Rheumatology. Philadelphia Lea & Febiger, 1960, pp. 250–273.
2. Lowman, E. W.: Arthritis: General Principles, Physical Medicine, Rehabilitation. Boston, Little, Brown & Company, 1959, 292 pp.
3. American Academy of Orthopaedic Surgeons: Measuring and Recording of Joint Motion. Everett, Massachusetts, Glenwood Press, 1963, 91 pp.

Suggested Reading for Additional Information

Anatomy of Joints

1. Barnett, C. H., Davies, D. V., and MacConaill, M. A.: Synovial Joints: Their Structure and Mechanics. Springfield, Illinois, Charles C Thomas, Publisher, 1961, 304 pp.
2. Gray, Henry: Anatomy of the Human Body. Ed. 27, Philadelphia, Lea & Febiger, 1959, 1458 pp.
3. Anson, B. J., and Maddock, W. G.: Callander's Surgical Anatomy. Ed. 4, Philadelphia, W. B. Saunders Company, 1958, 1105 pp.
4. Hollinshead, W. H.: Anatomy for Surgeons. New York, Paul B. Hoeber, Inc., 1956, vol. 2, 911 pp.
5. Grant, J. C. B.: An Atlas of Anatomy. Ed. 4, Baltimore, Williams & Wilkins Company, 1956, 634 Figs.
6. Grant, J. C. B.: A Method of Anatomy: Descriptive and Deductive. Ed. 5, Baltimore, Williams & Wilkins Company, 1952, 329 pp.
7. Morris, Henry: Human Anatomy. Ed. 11, New York, Blakiston Company, 1953, 1607 pp.
8. Brash, J. C.: Cunningham's Textbook of Anatomy. Ed. 9, London, Oxford University Press, 1951, 1559 pp.
9. Spalteholz, Werner: Hand-Atlas of Human Anatomy. Ed. 7, Philadelphia, J. B. Lippincott Company, 1943, vol. 1, 902 pp.

General Rheumatology

1. Committee of the American Rheumatism Association: Primer on the Rheumatic Diseases. J.A.M.A. *190*:127–140 (Oct. 12); 425–444 (Nov. 2); 509–530 (Nov. 9); 741–751 (Nov. 23) 1964.

2. Hollander, J. L.: Arthritis and Allied Conditions: A Textbook of Rheumatology. Ed. 6, Philadelphia, Lea & Febiger, 1960, 1306 pp.
3. Collins, D. H.: The Pathology of Articular and Spinal Diseases. Baltimore, Williams & Wilkins Company, 1950, 331 pp.
4. Talbott, J. H., and Ferrandis, R. M.: Collagen Diseases. New York, Grune & Stratton, Inc., 1956, 232 pp.
5. Short, C. L., Bauer, Walter, and Reynolds, W. E.: Rheumatoid Arthritis. Cambridge, Massachusetts, Harvard University Press, 1957, 457 pp.
6. McKusick, V. A.: Heritable Disorders of Connective Tissue. Ed. 2, St. Louis, C. V. Mosby Company, 1960, 333 pp.

CHAPTER TWO

TEMPOROMANDIBULAR JOINT

ESSENTIAL ANATOMY

INSPECTION

PALPATION

MOVEMENT AND RANGE OF MOTION

ESSENTIAL ANATOMY

The temporomandibular joint is formed by the fossa and the condyle of the mandible and the articular tubercle of the temporal bone. An articular disk of fibrocartilage divides the joint into two cavities each lined with synovial membrane. The synovial membrane is covered by a loose fibrous capsule which is strengthened laterally by the temporomandibular ligament. The paired temporomandibular joints are classified as a condylar joint since one bone (the mandible) articulates with the other (the skull) by two distinct articular surfaces or condyles. Thus each temporomandibular joint represents a condyle of the condylar joint, even though they are widely separated and are enclosed by different articular capsules.

INSPECTION

Swelling in this joint must be moderate or marked before it is apparent on inspection. If swelling is detectable, it appears as a rounded bulge in the area overlying the joint just anterior to the external auditory meatus (Fig. 2). Arthritis of the temporomandibular joint in young individuals may result in a disturbance of bone growth characterized by a shortened lower jaw (micrognathia; Fig. 3).

18

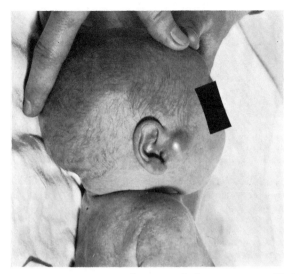

Figure 2.   Acute septic involvement of the temporomandibular joint due to staphylococcal infection in an infant.

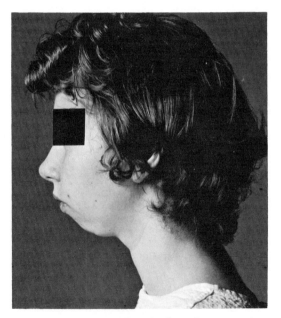

Figure 3.   Receding chin and underslung lower jaw (micrognathia) in a patient with juvenile rheumatoid arthritis involving the temporomandibular joint.

19

PALPATION

The joint can be located by placing the tip of the forefinger just anterior to the external auditory meatus and asking the patient to open his mouth. The tip of the examiner's finger then drops into an area overlying the joint proper. Moderate degrees of swelling in the joint prevent the fingertip from entering the depressed area overlying the joint. Swelling of marked degree may be palpable as a rounded, often fluctuant mass overlying the temporomandibular joint. By palpating the condyle and noting its location in the mandibular fossa with the patient's jaw closed, partially open, and wide open, the physician can determine various degrees of dislocation. Palpable or audible snapping or clicking of the temporomandibular joint occurs in many persons without evidence of arthritic disease. In the presence of palpable synovitis, local tenderness and warmth may be noted on palpation of the temporomandibular joint.

MOVEMENT AND RANGE OF MOTION

The temporomandibular joint permits three types of motion: opening and closing of the jaws, protrusion and retrusion of the mandible (anterior and posterior motion), and lateral or side-to-side motion.

Movement at each temporomandibular joint has two components. The inferior portion of the joint is formed by the mandibular condyle and articular disk and functions as a hinge joint, whereas the superior portion of the joint between the temporal bone and articular disk acts as a sliding joint, allowing both the disk and the mandible to glide forward, backward, and from side to side. When the jaws are opened and closed, motion, causing the mandible to rotate about a center of suspension slightly above the angle of the mandible, occurs in both portions of each joint. Anteroposterior movements of the mandible are performed mainly by the gliding action of the superior compartments, and lateral displacement of the jaw causes one articular disk to glide forward while the other remains in position. The grinding movements of chewing are produced by alternate movements in both compartments.

Vertical motion in this joint is determined most readily by measuring the space between the upper and lower incisor teeth with the patient's mouth open maximally. Care should be taken to keep the lower jaw somewhat protruded during this measurement since maximal opening of the mandible depends on adequate forward positioning of the lower jaw as well as on the degree of vertical motion. Normally, this distance will be about 3 to 6 cm. Lateral motion of the jaw is measured by having the patient partially open his mouth, protrude the lower jaw, and then move the lower jaw from side to side. Since the position of the mandible in the anteroposterior direction can cause considerable variation in the degree of lateral motion of the jaw, it is best to evaluate lateral motion with the jaw protruded as far as possible. The extent of lateral motion of the lower jaw is normally about 1 or 2 cm. Lateral motion may be lost earlier and to a greater degree than vertical motion. Finally, the patient is asked to protrude the lower jaw to see if it deviates to one side during protrusion.

Suggested Reading for Additional Information

1. Sarnat, B. G., and Laskin, D. M.: Diagnosis and Surgical Management of Diseases of the Temporomandibular Joint. Springfield, Illinois, Charles C Thomas, Publisher, 1962, 90 pp.
2. Schwartz, Laszlo: Disorders of the Temporomandibular Joint: Diagnosis, Management, Relation to Occlusion of Teeth. Philadelphia, W. B. Saunders Company, 1959, 471 pp.
3. Hollinshead, W. H.: Anatomy for Surgeons. New York, Paul B. Hoeber, Inc., 1954, vol. 1, pp. 358–360.

CHAPTER THREE

ACROMIOCLAVICULAR JOINT

ESSENTIAL ANATOMY

The acromioclavicular joint is a simple spheroidal joint formed by the lateral end of the clavicle and the medial margin of the acromion process of the scapula. There may or may not be a fibrocartilaginous articular disk in the joint cavity, but the joint is lined with synovial membrane. The joint is enveloped by a fibrous capsule that is strengthened by superior and inferior acromioclavicular ligaments. Often a subcutaneous bursa is located superficially over the acromioclavicular joint, but it rarely communicates with the joint cavity.

INSPECTION AND PALPATION

Although the acromioclavicular joint lies near the surface, localized swelling and tenderness in this area are best determined by palpation rather than by inspection, because of the close proximity of the joint to the prominence of the shoulder. First one acromioclavicular joint and then the other one is palpated with the examiner's fingertips and the joint on one side is compared with the joint on the other side. Palpation is best accomplished with the examiner in front of the patient and with the patient either sitting or standing. Localized tenderness and pain with movement confined to this area are observed more often than localized swelling is and are more significant findings since swelling in this region is difficult to localize accurately by inspection or palpation. Adduction of the patient's arm across his chest or shrugging of his shoulder may produce pain and help localize tenderness in disorders of the acromioclavicular joint.

MOVEMENT AND RANGE OF MOTION

This joint enables the scapula to move vertically when the shoulder girdle rises (shrugging the shoulders) and falls. It also enables the scapulae to rotate backward and forward on the clavicle. When the arm is raised above the head, the acromioclavicular joint participates in the movement of the scapula and the accompanying elevation of the shoulder. (Scapular movement accounts for most of the final 90 degrees of vertical motion when the arm is raised above the head.) However, actual measurements of the range of motion in the acromio-clavicular joint are not necessary in the usual rheumatologic examination of the joint.

Suggested Reading for Additional Information

Acromioclavicular and Sternoclavicular Joints

1. Hollinshead, W. H.: Anatomy for Surgeons. New York, Paul B. Hoeber, Inc., 1958, vol. 3, pp. 265–270.
2. DePalma, A. F.: Degenerative Changes in the Sternoclavicular and Acromio-clavicular Joints in Various Decades. Springfield, Illinois, Charles C Thomas, Publisher, 1957, 178 pp.
3. Moseley, H. F.: Shoulder Lesions. Ed. 2, New York, Paul B. Hoeber, Inc., 1953, 329 pp.
4. Codman, E. A.: The Shoulder. Boston, Thomas Todd Company, Printers, 1934, 513 pp.

CHAPTER FOUR

STERNOCLAVICULAR JOINT

ESSENTIAL ANATOMY

INSPECTION AND PALPATION

MOVEMENT AND RANGE OF MOTION

ESSENTIAL ANATOMY

The medial end of the clavicle articulates with the sternum and with the first costal cartilage to form the sternoclavicular joint on each side of the upper end of the manubrium. The sternoclavicular joint is a simple spheroidal joint. A fibrocartilaginous disk separates each joint into two separate cavities, the chondroclavicular and the chondrosternal. Both are lined with synovial membrane. A fibrous tissue capsule surrounds the entire joint and is strengthened by anterior and posterior sternoclavicular ligaments and the interclavicular ligament.

INSPECTION AND PALPATION

The sternoclavicular joint lies just beneath the skin, and redness and swelling in this area are easily seen when present. Synovitis of this joint may produce a smooth rounded swelling extending over the entire area (Fig. 4). With lesser degrees of synovitis the swelling may be more easily detected just lateral to the sternoclavicular joint in the depression between the clavicle and the first rib.

The chondroclavicular and chondrosternal components of the sternoclavicular joint are best palpated with the tips of the examiner's second and third fingers while comparing the two sternoclavicular joints. The consistency and location of swelling and the presence or absence of tenderness and local heat can be determined easily by palpation and by such comparison.

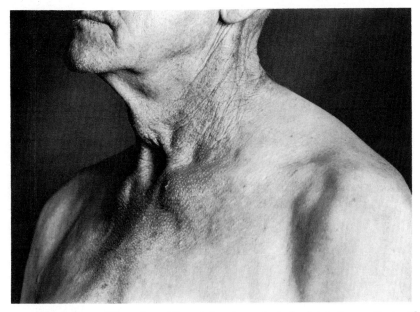

Figure 4.   Bilateral swelling of the sternoclavicular joints in a patient with rheumatoid arthritis.

MOVEMENT AND RANGE OF MOTION

The two sternoclavicular joints are the only points of articulation of the shoulder girdle with the trunk. Thus, in any motion of the shoulder girdle, there is motion of the sternoclavicular joint unless this joint is ankylosed. Discomfort may occur in the region of the sterno-clavicular joint on motion of the shoulder girdle, but measurement of motion of the sternoclavicular joint in degrees is not practicable.

Suggested Reading for Additional Information

Refer to references to Chapter 3, page 23.

CHAPTER FIVE

THE SHOULDER JOINT

ESSENTIAL ANATOMY

    Articular Capsule and Synovial Membrane
    The Rotator Cuff of the Shoulder
    Bursae

INSPECTION

PALPATION

    Rotator Cuff
    Articular Capsule, Synovial Membrane, and
       Glenohumeral Joint
    Bursae Adjacent to the Shoulder
    Bicipital Groove

MOVEMENT AND RANGE OF MOTION

REFERRED PAIN

ESSENTIAL ANATOMY

The shoulder or glenohumeral joint is a spheroidal or ball-and-socket joint formed by the articulation of the head of the humerus with the shallow glenoid cavity of the scapula (glenoid fossa). The shoulder joint allows considerable mobility of the arm and is enclosed by a group of powerful muscles and tendons which strengthen the joint. The joint is protected superiorly by an arch formed by the coracoid process, the acromion, and the coraco-acromial ligament. The shoulder girdle is formed by the scapula and the clavicle; they articulate with each other at the acromiclavicular joint. The main portion or body of the scapula is a large, flat, triangular bone which does not articulate with any portion of the skeleton other than the humerus and clavicle and is connected to the posterior aspect of the chest wall only by axio-appendicular muscles (Figs. 5 to 7).

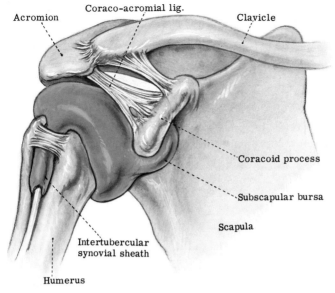

Acromion

Coraco-acromial lig.

Clavicle

Coracoid process

Subscapular bursa

Scapula

Intertubercular
synovial sheath

Humerus

Figure 5. Anterior aspect of shoulder joint showing the distribution of the distended synovial membrane of the glenohumeral joint and its relationship to adjacent bony structures. Synovial membrane, bursae, and synovial sheaths in this and subsequent drawings are shown in blue unless otherwise indicated.

Articular Capsule and Synovial Membrane

The fibrous articular capsule of the shoulder completely encircles the glenohumeral joint. It is attached superiorly (proximally) to the circumference of the glenoid cavity beyond the fibrocartilaginous rim of the glenoid labrum. Inferiorly (distally), it is attached to the anatomic neck of the humerus. The articular capsule is very loose and lax and allows the bones of the joint to separate from each other. The laxity of the articular capsule permits considerable freedom of motion which is characteristic of this joint. The articular capsule has two openings. One is an aperture in the attachment of the articular capsule to the humerus which allows the long tendon of the biceps muscle to enter the intertubercular (bicipital) groove of the humerus. The other aperture is located under the subscapular tendon and permits an extracapsular outpouching of the synovial membrane to function as a bursa for the subscapularis muscle.

The synovial membrane of the shoulder joint is situated beneath the fibrous capsule, tendons, muscles, and bursae. The inner surface of the articular capsule is lined by synovial membrane. The synovial membrane has two outpouchings, one of which (the subscapular portion) is actually extracapsular and functions as a bursa for the subscapularis muscle as mentioned. The other (the bicipital portion) extends along the intertubercular (bicipital) groove on the anterior aspect of the humerus and functions as a sheath for the tendon of the long head of the biceps muscle (Fig. 5).

The Rotator Cuff of the Shoulder

The broad, flat tendons of the supraspinatus, infraspinatus, and teres minor muscles insert into the greater tuberosity of the humerus, and the tendon of the subscapularis muscle inserts into the lesser tuberosity. Together these four muscles and tendons are termed the "rotator cuff of the shoulder." Prior to their insertions, each of the four tendons is incorporated in the fibrous cylindrical capsule that encloses the shoulder joint; consequently, the articular capsule is reinforced by these tendons. Reinforcement of the capsule is accomplished anteriorly by the subscapularis tendon, superiorly by the supraspinatus tendon, and posteriorly by the infraspinatus and the teres minor tendons.

Bursae

Overlying the tendinous and capsular cuff of the shoulder is the large *subacromial bursa* (Fig. 6). The lateral extension of this bursa is termed the "subdeltoid bursa" since it lies beneath the deltoid

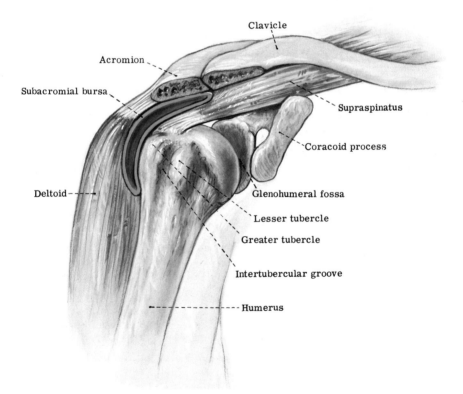

Figure 6.   Anterior aspect of the shoulder joint showing palpable landmarks and their relationship to the subacromial bursa.

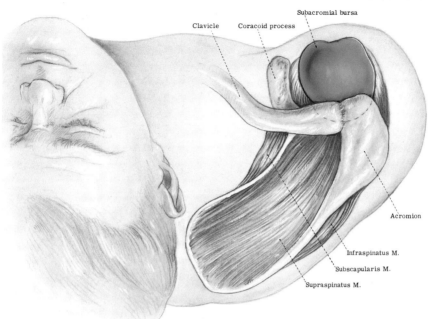

Clavicle   Coracoid process   Subacromial bursa

Acromion

Infraspinatus M.

Subscapularis M.

Supraspinatus M.

Figure 7.   The shoulder (glenohumeral) joint viewed from above showing bony landmarks and their relationship to the subacromial bursa.

muscle. The subacromial bursa facilitates movement of the greater tuberosity of the humerus beneath the acromion during abduction of the arm. Abduction of the shoulder compresses this bursa and also causes the acromion to impinge on the insertion of the supraspinatus tendon (Fig. 8). The subacromial bursa communicates with the joint cavity in approximately 20 to 33 per cent of individuals past middle age. Since the supraspinatus tendon forms the roof of the shoulder capsule and the floor of the subacromial bursa (Fig. 6), any tear of the tendon is likely to result in a communication between the bursa and the joint cavity.

The *subcoracoid bursa* lies between the capsule of the shoulder and the coracoid process. It may be separate from, or may communicate with, the subacromial bursa. Another small bursa, called the "subcutaneous acromial bursa," lies over the acromion process. Several other bursae occur about the shoulder; these may be significant anatomically but are relatively insignificant clinically.

INSPECTION

Inspection of the shoulders is performed with the patient's clothing removed at least to the level of the waist and if possible

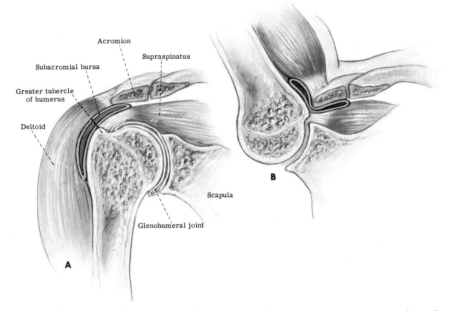

Figure 8. Relationship of subacromial bursa to supraspinatus muscle and acromion process. A. In position of adduction of humerus. In order to show this more clearly the synovial membrane of the glenohumeral joint is not shown in blue. B. In position of abduction of humerus the acromion impinges on the subacromial bursa and the insertion of the supraspinatus tendon.

with the patient either sitting or standing. Both shoulders are compared anteriorly and posteriorly for evidence of swelling and muscular atrophy or fasciculations over the trapezius, deltoid, scapular, and pectoral muscles. Atrophy of the supraspinatus and infraspinatus muscles is recognized as a lack of fullness in the respective superior and inferior scapular fossae (Fig. 9). Inequality or malposition of normal bony landmarks, such as the clavicle, acromion, coracoid process, or greater tuberosity of the humerus should be apparent by comparison of both sides. If the shoulder is dislocated anteriorly, the rounded lateral aspect of the shoulder is lost and appears flattened. Posterior dislocation of the shoulder, which is relatively rare, causes a flattening of the anterior aspect of the shoulder and sometimes produces a prominence of the humeral head, which can be seen over the posterior aspect of the shoulder in a thin individual.

A moderate to considerable amount of synovitis or fluid must be present in the glenohumeral joint to cause visible distention of the articular capsule. When present, this usually occurs over the anterior aspect of the joint (Fig. 10). Occasionally, intra-articular effusion may be detected in an individual with thin musculature as the result of fluid gravitating along the long head of the biceps in the intertubercular

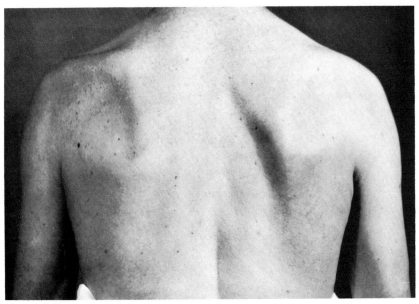

Figure 9.   Prominence of scapulae and atrophy of scapular, rhomboid, and serratus muscles in a patient with cervical radiculitis. Scapula is more prominent on the right, but the muscular atrophy is greater on the left side.

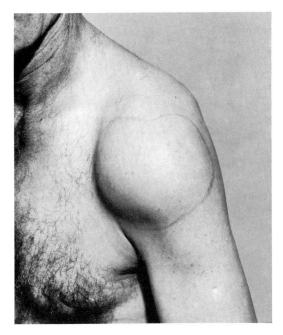

Figure 10.   Synovial cyst of left shoulder joint of patient with rheumatoid arthritis. Fluctuant, palpable portion of cyst is outlined in ink.

31

synovial sheath (Fig. 5) and causing abnormal fullness in this area. Swelling or distention of the subacromial bursa may produce localized fullness under the deltoid muscle which may be accentuated by partial abduction of the arm since part of the bursa is compressed in this position (Fig. 8). Effusion of the subacromial bursa may be due to localized disease of the bursa or may represent articular disease when the bursa communicates with the joint cavity. Occasionally distention of the subcoracoid bursa may cause a small bulge just lateral to the coracoid process, and distention of the subcutaneous acromial bursa may cause swelling localized to the region just above the acromio-clavicular joint.

Inspection and palpation are often combined in the examination of the shoulder.

PALPATION

Before the shoulder is examined by palpation, it is helpful to have the patient point out the area of maximal pain or tenderness by touching the involved shoulder with the hand of the uninvolved side. Since the patient cannot differentiate between referred pain to the shoulder and localized disease in the shoulder, the physician must utilize the examination (as well as the history) to establish the source and nature of pain in the shoulder. Pain originating in the shoulder joint must be demonstrable locally and reproducible by palpation or motion by the examiner when the patient can localize tenderness in order to differentiate it from pain referred to the shoulder because of extra-articular and potentially serious diseases (see p. 42). Sometimes the patient is unable to define a localized area of superficial tenderness and can only locate the area as "deep" in the general region of the shoulder. In such instances the patient's vague localization is of relatively little diagnostic value and the examiner must rely on evidence of localization obtained from the physical examination.

If possible, the patient is in either the sitting or the standing position during examination. Initially, the examiner can best evaluate abnormalities of the shoulder by positioning himself in front of the patient and palpating both shoulders for evidence of swelling, tenderness, local heat, muscle spasm, and atrophy. In this position with this routine he can compare the two shoulders easily. Then each shoulder can be examined from the side or posteriorly to obtain additional information.

A systematic examination of the shoulder includes palpation of the acromioclavicular joint (see p. 22), the rotator cuff, the region of the subacromial bursa, the intertubercular (bicipital) groove, and the anterior, lateral, and posterior aspects of the glenohumeral joint and the articular capsule. Palpation of the axilla for adenopathy and masses is also important.

Rotator Cuff

The posterior portion of the rotator cuff (tendons of infraspinatus and teres minor) is examined by having the patient adduct the arm across the chest and place his hand on the opposite shoulder. The examiner then stands in front of the patient and palpates the humeral head posteriorly with his thumb on the anterior aspect and with his fingers on the posterior aspect of the patient's shoulder; the posterior portion of the rotator cuff is then beneath the examiner's fingers. The anterior portion of the cuff (subscapularis tendon) is examined by placing the patient's arm in backward extension (drawn backward about 20 degrees from the axillary line while the arm is still in adduction) and by palpating it anteriorly over the humeral head. If the examiner stands behind the patient and places his fingers over the head of the humerus anteriorly while the patient internally rotates the arm by bringing his hand backward to a point between the scapulae, the superior portion of the rotator cuff (supraspinatus tendon) is then under the examiner's fingers and can be felt to move in this manner. During these maneuvers the examiner palpates the tendinous cuff for tenderness, swelling, firm nodular masses, or actual gaps (tears) in the cuff. Occasionally he can palpate a soft tender swelling which may represent the remaining proximal stub of a ruptured tendon attached to the humerus.

Degenerative lesions and abnormal calcium deposition in the rotator cuff frequently produce pain and tenderness over the upper portion of the humerus on the lateral aspect of the arm near the greater tuberosity. In contrast, bicipital lesions cause maximal tenderness over the anterior portion of the humerus in the region of the intertubercular (bicipital) groove.

Articular Capsule, Synovial Membrane, and Glenohumeral Joint

The fibrous articular capsule of the shoulder is so closely associated with the tendons of the rotator cuff that both of these structures must be palpated simultaneously since it is not possible to discriminate between them (as described in the section on palpation of the rotator cuff). If synovitis or effusion of the glenohumeral joint is detectable, a fluctuant distention is usually palpable, or warmth may be noticed over the anterior portion of the articular capsule and synovial membrane; however, the posterior portion of the capsule should also be palpated. Sometimes an effusion of the shoulder joint may cause palpable swelling along the bicipital extension of the synovial membrane in the intertubercular (bicipital) groove (Fig. 5). When the margins of the synovial membrane or articular capsule are palpable, a moderate to considerable amount of synovitis or effusion is present since mild degrees of synovitis of the shoulder joint are not palpable.

Bursae Adjacent to the Shoulder

Inflammation or irritation of the subacromial (subdeltoid) bursa may result in palpable swelling, tenderness, and warmth of the upper portion of the arm in the region of the deltoid muscle and just distal to the acromion process. Inflammation is usually associated with degenerative lesions or calcium deposition in the rotator cuff. Since a communication between the articular cavity and the subacromial bursa may occur, effusion of the joint may sometimes be detected by swelling and distention of the subacromial bursa.

Bicipital Groove

Inflammation of the synovial sheath or the tendon of the long head of the biceps muscle (bicipital tenosynovitis) produces pain in the region of the intertubercular (bicipital) groove. The pain may extend along the biceps muscle into the forearm. The condition is best detected by palpation over the intertubercular (bicipital) groove which extends along the anterior aspect of the upper end of the humerus (Fig. 5). Palpation is performed while the patient's arm and forearm are rotated externally and with the examiner's fingers placed anteriorly over the groove to localize pain and to ascertain any tenderness, crepitus, or swelling in this region. Sometimes tenderness in this area may be increased considerably by rolling the bicipital tendon under the finger tips. If desired, the examiner may place his thumb posteriorly behind the arm to stabilize the examining fingers. The bicipital tendon and groove on the opposite side are palpated for comparison.

If the patient's elbow is held at his side and flexed at a right angle while the forearm is supinated against resistance supplied by the examiner's hand, pain will often be produced in the bicipital groove if tendinitis or tenosynovitis is present (Yergason's sign). Another maneuver useful in localizing involvement to the bicipital tendon is performed by passively extending the elbow while the patient's hand and forearm are in the position of supination and the shoulder is passively moved posteriorly into a hyperextended position. A positive response to this maneuver is indicated by the localization of pain in the bicipital groove. Flexion of the forearm against resistance applied by the examiner or active anterior flexion of the extended arm against resistance also may cause pain over the anterior portion of the arm and along the biceps tendon if an abnormality of the bicipital tendon is present.

34

MOVEMENT AND RANGE OF MOTION

Motion of the upper extremity on the trunk is normally a combination of movement of the shoulder girdle and the shoulder joint. The ball-and-socket shoulder joint is capable of a wide variety of movements. It permits flexion (forward movement of the arm), extension (dorsal flexion or backward movement of the arm), abduction (elevation of the arm from the side), adduction (lowering the arm to the side), rotation, and circumduction. The movements of the shoulder girdle as a whole on the chest wall include elevation (raising or shrugging the shoulder girdle above the normal resting position), depression (downward motion of the shoulder girdle below the normal resting position), protrusion (advancement of the shoulder girdle in front of the coronal plane), retraction (backward motion of the shoulder girdle behind the coronal plane), and circumduction.

Elevation of the arm from the side of the body (abduction) up over the head is accomplished by the combined movement of the shoulder joint and rotation of the scapula on the chest wall. This movement also is associated with motion of the sternoclavicular and acromioclavicular joints. Although there has been a tendency to separate active abduction of the arm into two distinct parts consisting of elevation of the arm to the horizontal position (using the glenohumeral joint) and raising of the arm from the horizontal position overhead (using scapulothoracic motion), such a distinction is artificial since both joints participate throughout abduction of the arm. As active normal elevation of the arm begins, only slight motion of the scapula occurs until the arm is in about 30 degrees of abduction. Thereafter rotation of the scapula becomes more marked as the arm is raised over the head; after about 30 degrees of abduction, however, the glenohumeral joint contributes approximately twice as much to abduction as scapular motion does. The relatively active normal movement of the shoulder joint and the scapulothoracic articulation may vary considerably in different individuals during abduction of the arm. When motion of the glenohumeral joint is limited by disease or muscle spasm, the individual may compensate by elevation of the entire shoulder girdle, using a hunching motion in an effort to abduct the arm more completely (Fig. 11).

Four simple maneuvers may be used as an introductory or screening procedure for evaluation of the range of motion of the shoulder:

1. The patient is asked to extend both elbows fully (at the sides of the body) and then to move both the arms upward in wide vertical arcs (forward flexion or forward elevation) in an effort to touch the palmar surface of both hands together above the head (Fig. 12).

2. The patient is asked to touch both hands on the top of his

35

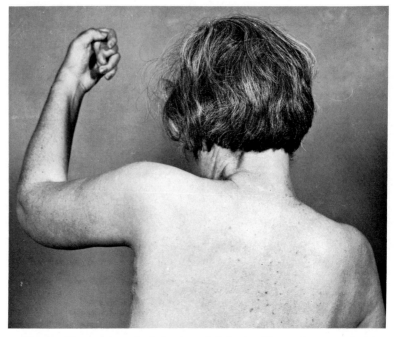

Figure 11.   Limited abduction of left shoulder and severe flexion contractures of the fingers in a patient with shoulder-hand syndrome.

head with the elbows flexed and the upper extremities moving in a horizontal arc posteriorly.

3. The patient is asked to raise each extended arm above his head in a wide sideways arc in the coronal plane of the body (abduction), finally attempting to touch the palmar surface of his hands together above his head with arms and forearms fully extended (Fig. 13).

4. The patient is asked to rotate his arm internally behind his back and place the back of his hand as high as possible between the scapulae (Fig. 14).

The relative contributions of scapular and humeral motions are easily observed during these maneuvers by inspection or palpation or both of the patient from behind. Scapular motion also may be indicated by the degree of elevation of the shoulder. If this initial survey shows limitation of motion, the range of motion of the glenohumeral joint then may be examined in more detail.

Relatively little external rotation of the humerus is required when the arm is elevated over the head by forward flexion, whereas external rotation of about 180 degrees occurs when elevation of the arm is performed by abduction in a sideways arc over the head touching the palmar surface of the hands together. Thus, lesions affecting the rotating musculature of the humerus or the rotator cuff may cause

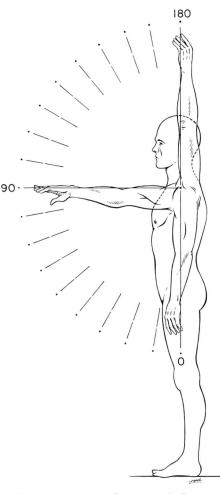

Figure 12. Forward flexion of extended arm. This examination may be performed on each upper extremity separately or on both together. In the latter instance, the patient touches the palmar surface of both hands together over the head.

pain, muscle spasm, or limitation of motion on abduction of the arm while the range of forward flexion of the arm may remain relatively normal. Forward flexion of the arm is often a more reliable indication of the extent of shoulder motion than abduction is, since patients with muscle spasm and misuse of antagonist muscles may either restrict abduction of the arm or elevate the arm slowly, whereas they are able to accomplish the forward flexion with relative ease.

The motions which are of most value in the evaluation of the normal function of the glenohumeral joint are internal rotation, external rotation, and abduction. For accurate measure of glenohumeral abduction, motion of the scapula should be prevented. This is best accomplished if the examiner grasps the inferior portion of the scapula and holds it firmly in place with one hand while he passively and slowly abducts the patient's arm with his other hand and forearm. The muscles of the abducted arm must be relaxed. This can be accomplished by

37

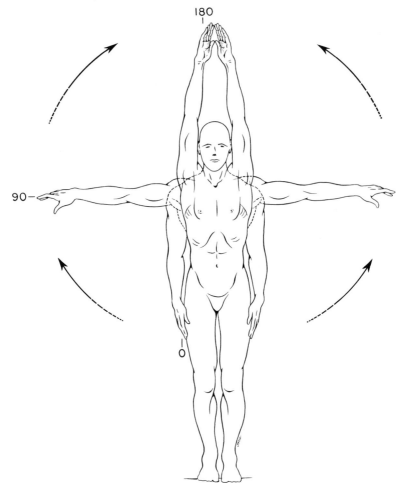

Figure 13. Abduction of both extended arms in a sideways arc in the coronal plane of the body, touching the palmar surface of the hands together above the head.

allowing the patient's arm and forearm to rest on the arm and forearm of the examiner while the examiner's arm is slowly elevated. When the patient or examiner detects the appearance of muscle spasm, the examiner should temporarily stop the motion and ask the patient to press his elbow slightly downward onto the examiner's arm. This will relax the spasm at least temporarily and permit further attempts at passive abduction. If the scapula is adequately stabilized during this procedure, there should be no elevation of the shoulder or shoulder girdle. The scapula can be partially but satisfactorily stabilized by exerting downward and restricting pressure on the acromion to prevent elevation of the shoulder girdle. The normal range of abduction of the glenohumeral joint under these circumstances is about 90 degrees or slightly more from the 0 degree position with the arm resting at the side (Fig. 15).

Since the scapula normally moves during rotation of the shoulder and thus is a component of useful shoulder function, the entire shoulder girdle may be allowed to participate in measurement of rotation. Rotation of the arm is best demonstrated when the examiner places himself at the side of the patient who is either sitting or standing. Then, with the patient's elbow bent at a right angle and the forearm horizontal (0 degrees; Fig. 16), the forearm is moved upward (external rotation of the shoulder) and downward (internal rotation of the shoulder). The normal range is about 90 degrees of internal rotation and 90 degrees of external rotation as is shown in Figure 16.

Tears of the rotator cuff of the shoulder characteristically produce inability or limitation of active abduction of the arm from the side. Sometimes an individual with a partial tear of the rotator cuff can initiate abduction of the arm partway but is unable to raise the arm to a horizontal position. If the patient's arm is passively abducted to a horizontal position by the examiner, the patient then may have little or no difficulty in raising his arm over his head or lowering his arm

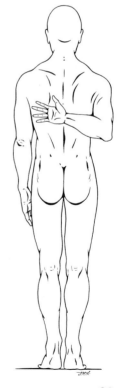

Figure 14. Position of right hand and arm placed behind the back in test of range of internal rotation of right shoulder. The patient should place his hand as high as possible between the scapulae, and the range of motion in the two shoulders is compared.

to a horizontal position, but if the arm is lowered below a 90-degree angle, it may fall suddenly to the patient's side. Some individuals can hold the involved arm in a horizontal position when it is abducted by the examiner or by the patient's uninvolved arm, but the ability to maintain the arm in abduction against resistance applied in a downward direction by the examiner is distinctly impaired. Attempted abduction of the arm by a patient with a tear of the rotator cuff may produce a characteristic hunching motion of the shoulder since the rotator cuff is unable to stabilize the humeral head adequately within the glenoid fossa of the scapula (Fig. 17).

Degenerative lesions of the rotator cuff often cause pain that starts when the arm is in about 70 degrees of abduction and disappears after the arm is raised above 100 degrees of abduction since the acromion process tends to impinge on the rotator cuff and subacromial bursa between these degrees of motion in abduction (Fig. 8).

When secondary adhesive capsulitis (frozen shoulder) has developed, the cause of the original abnormality is often obscured. Initial physical examination of the shoulder alone may not permit differentiation of tears of the musculotendinous cuff, reflex dystrophy, rheumatoid arthritis, and other types of involvement of the shoulder that can result in a frozen shoulder.

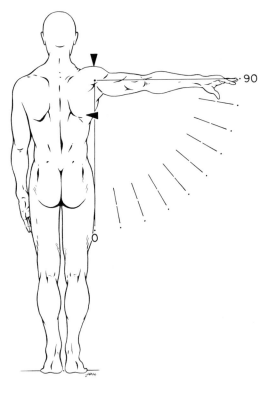

Figure 15. Range of abduction of the glenohumeral joint with the scapula and shoulder girdle stabilized in the areas marked by the black triangles. See text for details.

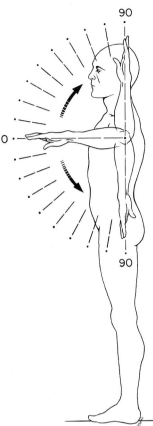

Figure 16. Range of internal and external rotation of the shoulder. With elbow bent at a right angle and forearm held horizontally, the forearm is moved upward for external rotation and downward for internal rotation. This examination also can be done while the patient is supine.

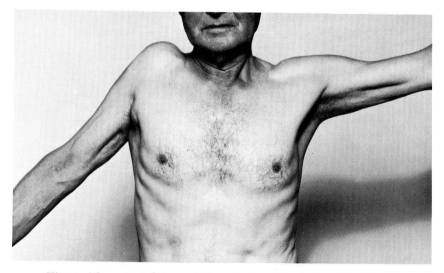

Figure 17. Partial tear of the rotator cuff of the right shoulder with limitation of abduction of the arm and a characteristic hunched position of the involved shoulder as compared with abduction of the unaffected left shoulder.

41

REFERRED PAIN

Many disease processes in areas other than the shoulder may cause pain in the shoulder region and can be confused with involvement of the shoulder or adjacent structures. Cardiac disease, involvement of the pleura, and hiatal hernia, all may produce pain that is referred to the shoulder. Subphrenic inflammation may irritate the inferior portion of the diaphragm and produce referred pain and tenderness in the region of the neck and shoulder. Diseases of the cervical portion of the spinal column, nerve roots, or peripheral nerves in the upper extremity are frequent extraneous sources of shoulder pain and disability. Sometimes these extraneous sources of shoulder pain may cause difficulty in the recognition and interpretation of symptoms in the region of the shoulder.

Suggested Reading for Additional Information

1. Moseley, H. F.: Disorders of the Shoulder, Ciba Clin. Symposia. 2:251 (Oct.) 1950.
2. Moseley, H. F.: Shoulder Lesions. Ed. 2, New York, Paul B. Hoeber, Inc., 1953, 329 pp.
3. Hollinshead, W. H.: Anatomy for Surgeons. New York, Paul B. Hoeber, Inc., 1958, vol. 3, pp. 263–281.
4. Bateman, J. E.: The Shoulder and Environs. St. Louis, C V. Mosby Company, 1955, 539 pp.
5. Codman, E. A.: The Shoulder. Boston, Thomas Todd Company, Printers, 1934, 513 pp.
6. Steinbrocker, Otto: The Painful Shoulder. In Hollander, J. L.: Arthritis and Allied Conditions. Ed. 6, Philadelphia, Lea & Febiger, 1960, pp. 1181–1227.
7. American Academy of Orthopaedic Surgeons: Measuring and Recording of Joint Motion. Everett, Massachusetts, Glenwood Press, 1963, 91 pp.

CHAPTER SIX

THE ELBOW

ESSENTIAL ANATOMY

The elbow (articulatio cubiti) is a hinge joint formed by the humero-ulnar, radiohumeral, and proximal radio-ulnar articulations. Thus the elbow actually is composed of three bony articulations, the principal one of which is the humero-ulnar. All of these bony junctions are enclosed by the articular capsule in a common synovial articular cavity. Thus, the synovial membrane of the elbow is relatively extensive. It is attached at the margin of the articular surface of the humerus and is reflected upward, lining the coronoid and olecranon fossae. It is reflected downward from this area to its attachment at the margin of the articular surfaces of the ulna and radius. There are three masses of fat between the synovial membrane and the overlying capsule; the largest lies over the olecranon fossa; the others lie over the coronoid fossa and the radial fossa. Since the synovial membrane is usually palpable only posteriorly, only the posterior aspect of the elbow is illustrated in Figure 18. The articular capsule is thickened laterally and medially to form the radial collateral and ulnar collateral ligaments. The para-olecranon grooves are the spaces between the olecranon process of the ulna and the medial and lateral epicondyles of the humerus.

One large bursa (olecranon) and several small bursae lie about the elbow. The latter are not uniformly present, and neither the olecranon nor the other bursae communicate with the joint cavity under normal conditions.

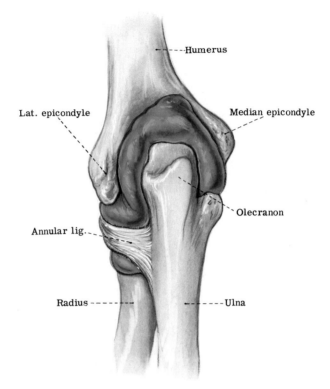

Figure 18.   Posterior aspect of elbow joint showing radius and ulna in extension and distribution of synovial membrane in distention.

INSPECTION

The elbows are best inspected while the patient is either sitting or standing. When this is not possible, the elbow of a patient in a supine position is examined by raising the shoulder forward 10 to 20 degrees and placing the arm across the patient's chest in as comfortable a position as possible. Medial and lateral deviations of the forearm on the arm are called "cubitus varus" and "cubitus valgus," respectively. When subluxation of the elbow occurs, the forearm is usually dislocated posteriorly in relation to the humerus (Fig. 19). Swelling and redness of the olecranon bursa are easily observed because of the close proximity of this bursa to the skin (Fig. 20). Common sites for subcutaneous nodules are in the olecranon bursa and along the extensor or most exposed surface of the ulna distal to the olecranon process (Fig. 21). When there is effusion or synovial thickening in the joint, the condition is usually first apparent as a bulge or fullness in the para-olecranon grooves on each side of the olecranon process (Fig. 22).

44

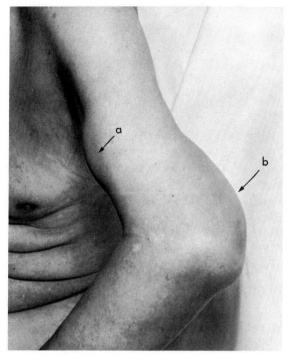

Figure 19.   Charcot's arthropathy of left elbow of a patient with tabes dorsalis showing severe subluxation and deformity. The humerus protrudes anteriorly (a) and the ulna posteriorly (b) above the level of the elbow.

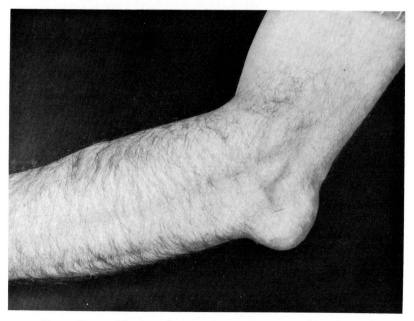

Figure 20.   Olecranon bursitis in a patient with tophaceous gout.

45

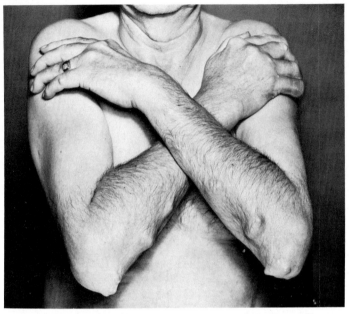

Figure 21. Subcutaneous nodules on the extensor surface of both fore-arms and hands in a patient with rheumatoid arthritis.

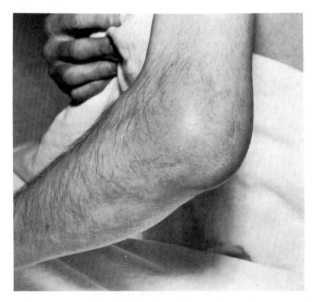

Figure 22. Acute gouty arthritis of the elbow showing swelling of the synovial membrane and perisynovial tissues on the posterior aspect of the joint.

PALPATION

Synovial Membrane

The elbow joint may be palpated with the patient in either the supine or sitting position, but the elbow should be as relaxed as possible. Irrespective of the position of the patient, the examiner will use his left hand to give firm support to the left forearm of the patient while his right thumb and fingers palpate the left elbow. The right elbow is examined in the same fashion except that the examiner palpates with his left thumb and fingers and uses his right hand to support the forearm. As shown in Figure 23, the thumb is placed over the lateral para-olecranon groove and the forefinger or middle finger or both are placed over the medial para-olecranon groove. These spaces are best palpated with the patient's elbow flexed about 70 degrees from the position of complete extension and with the muscles relaxed. Synovial thickening or joint effusion or both are more often palpable in the medial than in the lateral para-olecranon groove but should be discernible on palpation in both because of the anatomic distribution of the synovial membrane in this joint (Fig. 18). The pressure of the examining fingers and thumb should be varied while these digits palpate the para-olecranon grooves. A soft, boggy, or fluctuant fullness in both grooves indicates synovial thickening or effusion or both and can be differentiated from the more solid consistency of the adjacent fat pads and other soft tissues. Local heat or redness, if present, often extends beyond the confines of the synovial membrane. Slowly extending the patient's arm while the examiner keeps his thumb and fingers in the para-olecranon grooves often helps the examiner to identify synovitis. The synovial membrane may bulge under the palpating thumb or fingers as the forearm is extended. This maneuver also helps the examiner distinguish tendons, muscles, fat pads, and ligaments from the synovial membrane in this area. Occasionally the differentiation of synovial thickening from effusion may be suggested by palpation of the synovial membrane over the bony margins of the radiohumeral joint posteriorly.

The elbow is a common site of synovitis, but this involvement is often overlooked. In the detection of synovitis by physical examination it is particularly helpful to compare the physical findings of a suspected abnormal joint with those of a normal joint. Synovitis of the elbow also is commonly associated with limitation of extension of the joint.

Other Tissues

The *olecranon bursa* can be easily palpated for fluid, swelling, tenderness, local heat, consistency, loose bodies, and nodules. Nodules,

47

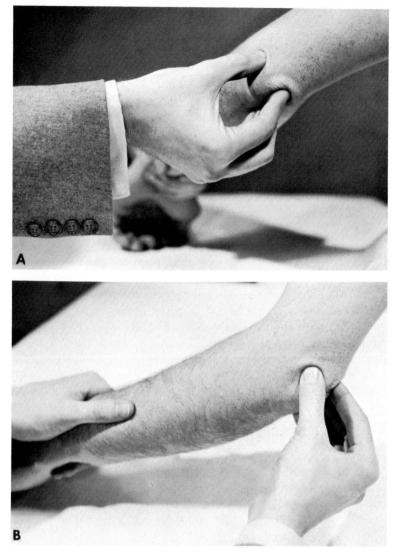

Figure 23. Palpation for synovial thickening or effusion of left elbow. A. Posterior view. B. Side view. The examiner's left hand is supporting the forearm with the elbow flexed about 70 degrees from the position of complete extension. The examiner's right thumb and fingers are used to palpate between the lateral and medial edges of the olecranon process and the humeral epicondyles. See text for details.

loose bodies, and tenderness are most apparent with the elbow fully flexed, whereas the bursa and adjacent tissues may be palpated best between the examiner's thumb and second finger with the patient's elbow extended. If the olecranon bursa is enlarged, the bursa may or may not be fixed to the underlying olecranon process.

48

Subcutaneous nodules may be large enough to be seen, but some that are not large enough to be visible can be palpated when the examiner runs his finger along the extensor surface of the ulna. Nodules are detected as raised, firm, nontender nodes on the extensor surface of the ulna in or distal to the olecranon bursa. The overlying skin and subcutaneous tissues can be moved freely over a subcutaneous nodule, but the mobility of the nodule depends on its location. When a nodule is in the olecranon bursa, it is relatively more movable than when it is in the subcutaneous tissues or affixed to the periosteum. Slight bony irregularities of the ulnar surface may be present in this area and are not abnormal.

The *medial and lateral epicondyles* of the humerus and the head of the radius and the tendinous attachments of muscles to these structures are common sites of inflammation, pain, or localized tenderness ("tennis elbow" or "epicondylitis"). The ulnar nerve and groove also can be palpated for indication of thickening, irregularity, and tenderness.

Swelling of the articular capsule occasionally may be detected by deep palpation of the antecubital space, but swelling in such instances is usually evident and more easily detected by the posterior examination of the elbow as described.

MOVEMENT AND RANGE OF MOTION

The position of complete extension of the elbow is designated here as 0 degrees. A few individuals normally lack 5 to 10 degrees of full extension, and others may have 5 to 10 degrees of hyperextension. When the joint is flexed, the angle between the arm and forearm normally is 160 to 150 degrees of flexion from the extended position (Fig. 24). The movements of flexion and extension occur in the humero-ulnar

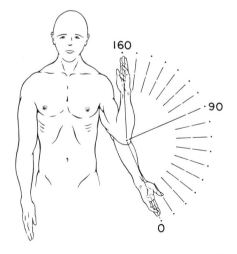

Figure 24. Range of normal flexion and extension of the elbow.

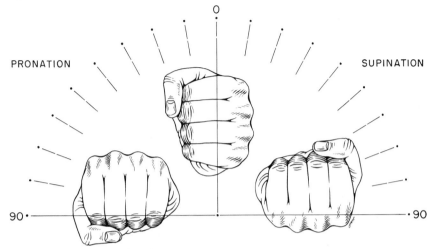

PRONATION   SUPINATION

O

90   90

Figure 25.   Normal range of pronation and supination of the hand and forearm. In this diagram the fingers are flexed to form a fist, but the examination can be made with the patient's fingers extended or semiflexed.

and radiohumeral joints. Pronation and supination of the hand and forearm involve motion of both radio-ulnar joints (at the elbow and the wrist) and the radiohumeral joint. Normally, these joints allow approximately 180 degrees of movement that can be divided into about 90 degrees of pronation and about 90 degrees of supination from a position midway between the two extremes (Fig. 25).

Suggested Reading for Additional Information

1. Anson, B. J., and Maddock, W. G.: Callander's Surgical Anatomy. Ed. 4, Philadelphia, W. B. Saunders Company, 1958, pp. 837–858.
2. Hollinshead, W. H.: Anatomy for Surgeons. New York, Paul B. Hoeber, Inc., 1958, vol. 3, pp. 379–389.
3. Smith, F. M.: Surgery of the Elbow. Springfield, Illinois, Charles C Thomas, Publisher, 1954, 340 pp.

CHAPTER SEVEN

THE WRIST AND CARPAL JOINTS

ESSENTIAL ANATOMY

Joints and Synovial Membranes

Wrist or Radiocarpal Articulation. This joint is formed proximally by the distal end of the radius and the articular disk and

51

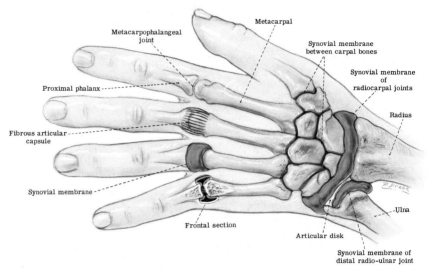

Figure 26. Relationship of the synovial membranes of the wrist, carpal, and metacarpophalangeal joints to adjacent bony and surface landmarks.

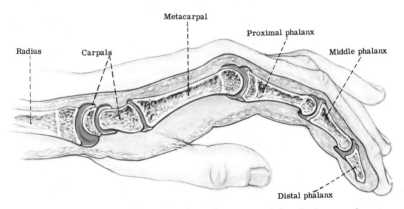

Figure 27. Sagittal section through wrist and hand showing location of synovial membranes. Note that the synovial membrane extends farther proximally than distally at the metacarpophalangeal and interphalangeal joints.

distally by a row of carpal bones, the navicular, the lunate, and the triangular (Fig. 26). The articular disk joins the radius to the ulna and separates the distal end of the ulna from the wrist joint proper. The wrist joint is surrounded by a capsule and supported by ligaments. The synovial membrane lines the inner surface of the articular capsule. The capsule and underlying synovial membrane are loose, especially over the dorsum of the wrist where the distal ends of the radius and ulna lie near the surface under the skin.

Distal Radio-ulnar Joint. This joint is adjacent to the radiocarpal joint (wrist joint) but usually is not a part of it since the articular disk divides these joints into two separate cavities (Fig. 26). The synovial membrane loosely lines the deep surface of the articular capsule and internal ligaments and bulges upward between the radius and ulna beyond the level of the articular surfaces.

Midcarpal Joint. The midcarpal joint is formed by the junction of the proximal and distal rows of carpal bones. It permits some flexion and extension and a slight amount of rotation. The midcarpal and carpometacarpal articular cavities often communicate and are lined with synovial membrane which covers the deep surfaces of the intercarpal ligaments and the surrounding capsule (Figs. 26 and 27).

Tendons and Synovial Sheaths of the Wrist and Hand; the Median Nerve

The synovial tendon sheaths of the wrist and hand will be discussed together.

Flexor Tendons. The long flexor tendons of the muscles of the forearm are enclosed in a common flexor tendon sheath (sometimes called the "ulnar bursa") which begins at the level of the wrist and extends to the midpalm. The tendon sheath of the flexor pollicis longus may be completely separate or may join the sheath of the common flexor tendon (Fig. 28). Part of the common flexor tendon sheath lies in a fibro-osseous canal (carpal tunnel) which is bounded anteriorly (palmar aspect) by the flexor retinaculum (transverse carpal ligament) and posteriorly (dorsal aspect) by the carpal bones and ligaments on the floor of the canal.

The flexor retinaculum is crossed anteriorly by the palmaris longus tendon and anteromedially by the ulnar nerve, ulnar artery, and ulnar vein. The latter three structures may have additional connective tissue covering them anteriorly (the volar carpal ligament or superficial part of the transverse carpal ligament), but this additional connective tissue is not involved in the production of the carpal tunnel syndrome.

Median Nerve. This nerve also runs through the carpal tunnel. It lies between the anterior surface of the common flexor tendon sheath and the flexor retinaculum and may be compressed by the firm unyielding flexor retinaculum if swelling or edema occurs in this region (Fig. 28).

The tendon sheath of the fifth finger is usually continuous with the common flexor tendon sheath, whereas the common flexor tendon sheath covering the tendons of the second (index), third (middle), and fourth (ring) fingers ends at midpalm. The flexor tendons then continue distally without a tendon sheath until covered individually by their respective digital synovial sheaths (Fig. 28).

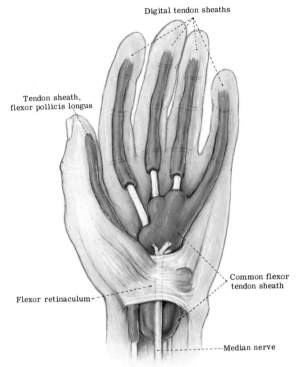

Digital tendon sheaths

Tendon sheath,
flexor pollicis longus

Common flexor
tendon sheath

Flexor retinaculum

Median nerve

Figure 28.   Anterior (palmar) aspect of the wrist and digits showing the distribution of the synovial sheaths of the flexor tendons. The median nerve lies between the anterior surface of the common flexor tendon sheath and the flexor retinaculum where it is subject to compression by the firm unyielding retinaculum if swelling occurs in this region.

Palmar Aponeurosis.   The palmar aponeurosis (fascia) begins at the level of the retinaculum as the apex of a triangle which fans out into the central portion of the palm. The apex of the aponeurosis is a direct continuation of the tendon of the palmaris longus. The central portion has thickened bands which lie over the flexor tendons and extend into the digits. The four bands to the second (index), third (middle), fourth (ring), and fifth (little) fingers are thicker and more constant than the one to the thumb.

Extensor Tendons.   The extensor tendons of the forearm pass through six fibro-osseous tunnels on the dorsum of the wrist. These tunnels are bound superficially by the extensor retinaculum (dorsal carpal ligament) and on the deep surface by the carpal bones and ligaments. Each tunnel is lined with a synovial sheath which extends about an inch proximally and distally from the extensor retinaculum (Fig. 29). The long abductor and short extensor tendons of the thumb pass through the most radial of the six fibro-osseous tunnels. These tendons pass the prominence of the radial styloid process and thus

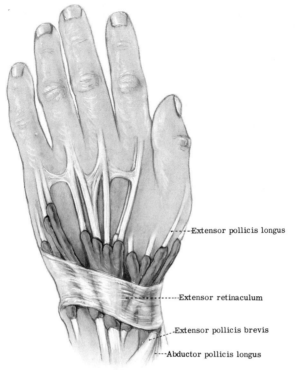

Extensor pollicis longus

Extensor retinaculum

Extensor pollicis brevis

Abductor pollicis longus

Figure 29. Posterior (dorsal) aspect of the wrist showing the distribution of the synovial sheaths of the extensor tendons. The extensor pollicis brevis and the abductor pollicis longus, the principal tendons involved in stenosing tenosynovitis at the radial styloid process, are identified.

are subject to particular friction and trauma at this site. A triangular depression over the dorsolateral aspect of the wrist which is visible when the thumb is extended and abducted is known as the anatomic "snuffbox." The long abductor and short extensor tendons of the thumb form the radial boundary, the long extensor tendon of the thumb forms the medial boundary, and the radial styloid process lies on the floor of the anatomic "snuffbox." The long extensor tendon of the thumb is particularly vulnerable to wear and fraying because it functions repeatedly over bony prominences. This tendon passes through a bony groove on the medial aspect of the dorsal tubercle of Lister where angulation caused by dorsiflexion or radial deviation may pull the tendon around a rough edge and also predispose to rupture.

INSPECTION

Swelling of the Wrist

Swelling of the wrist may be localized or diffuse (Figs. 30 and 31). Localized synovial swellings on the dorsum of the wrist may re-

55

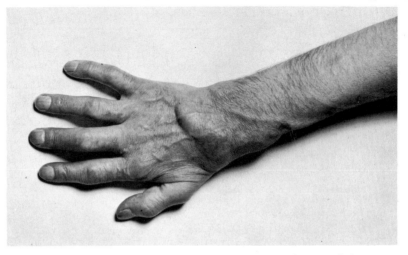

Figure 30. Cystic synovial outpouching on the dorsum of the wrist associated with tenosynovitis in a patient with rheumatoid arthritis.

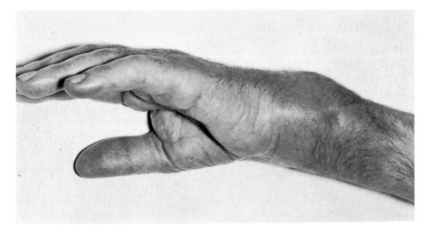

Figure 31. Diffuse swelling, edema, and induration accompanying staphylococcal arthritis of the wrist.

semble cysts and result from synovial outpouchings of tendon sheaths or from outpouchings of the synovial membrane lining the wrist joint. In the latter instance the synovial swelling lies adjacent to the extensor tendons; when articular synovial swelling is seen on the volar aspect of the wrist, it lies adjacent to the flexor tendons. Similar cystic synovial swelling may arise from the tendon sheaths in the hand and may be found anywhere in the hand, but it will be within the confines of the tendon sheath or sheaths involved.

    Ganglion. The term "ganglion" (plural: ganglia or ganglions) is used commonly to describe a cystic enlargement which characteristi-

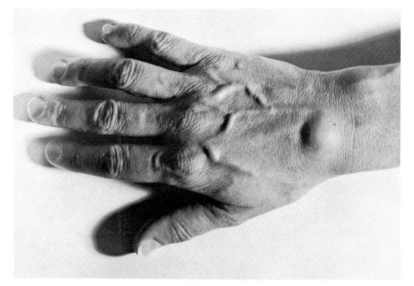

Figure 32.　　Ganglion or small cystic swelling on dorsum of right hand just distal to the wrist joint.

cally occurs on the dorsal surface of the wrist along tendon sheaths or joint capsules or between the tendons of the common extensors of the digits and the radial extensors at the base of the second metacarpal bone (Fig. 32). Other common sites for ganglia are the anatomic "snuffbox" at the base of the thumb on the dorsal aspect of the hand and on the radial side of the volar aspect of the wrist. Ganglia also may arise from the tendon sheaths of the flexor tendons over the proximal phalanges of the fingers, usually just beyond the distal palmar crease.

A ganglion may result from a localized herniation of synovial membrane from a joint or tendon sheath or may be regarded as a benign synovial tumor (Fig. 32). In either instance it has a synovial lining membrane resembling that of diarthrodial joints, tendon sheaths, or bursae. Ganglia contain a thick mucoid or semisolid material and may vary in size from those that are only barely visible on inspection to those that are several centimeters in diameter. They usually cause relatively few, if any, symptoms other than localized swelling and mild discomfort with motion, but they can become tender and painful when distended.

Deformity of the Wrist and Function of the Hand

Proper positioning of the wrist is essential for adequate function of the hand. When the wrist is flexed (palmar), much of the power of flexion in the fingers is lost. If the wrist is ankylosed or partially

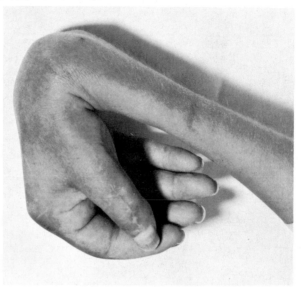

Figure 33. Ankylosis of the wrist in extreme flexion, resulting in a practically useless hand of a patient with severe rheumatoid arthritis.

fixed in flexion, the hand loses some of its usefulness because in this position the extensor tendons of the digits tend to extend the metacarpophalangeal joints and the thumb is extended and abducted, flattening this portion of the hand and making it difficult or impossible for the thumb to oppose the fingers (Fig. 33). At the same time, the interphalangeal joints become extended unless flexion contractures of the fingers have occurred. This is in contrast to the functional position of the hand when the wrist is partially extended (dorsiflexion); in this instance, the fingers and metacarpophalangeal joints can be flexed and the thumb positioned for opposing the fingers, producing useful hand function.

Other Abnormalities of the Wrist and Hand

In the usual deformity associated with thickening and contracture of the palmar aponeurosis (Dupuytren's contracture), the involved fingers are drawn into flexion contractures, first at the metacarpophalangeal joint, followed by flexion of the proximal interphalangeal joint. The fourth digit or ring finger is involved earliest, then the fifth and third digits in that order. The second and first digits are rarely affected. The skin may be irregularly bound down to the involved areas of the aponeurosis (Fig. 34).

Atrophy of thenar muscles suggests interference with the motor function of the median nerve at the wrist (carpal tunnel syndrome; Fig. 35). Abnormal dorsolateral prominence of the ulna indicates subluxa-

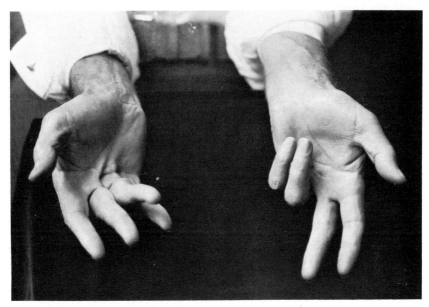

Figure 34. Dupuytren's contractures in both hands showing flexion contractures of the fourth and fifth digits of the left hand and less severe contractures in the third, fourth, and fifth digits of the right hand. Note the puckering of palmar skin and the presence of bands extending from the concavity of the palm to the proximal interphalangeal joints of the third and fourth digits of the right hand.

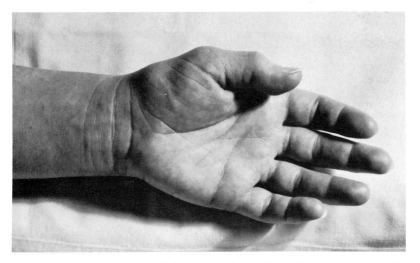

Figure 35. Atrophy of thenar muscles resulting from compression of the median nerve in the carpal tunnel (carpal tunnel syndrome).

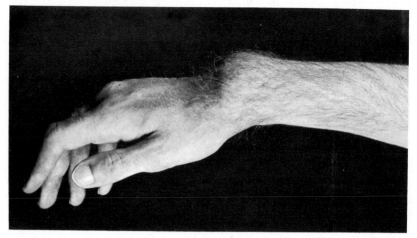

Figure 36.   Subluxation of wrist with prominence of the dorsally protruding ulna resulting from severe rheumatoid arthritis. Moderate synovitis of wrist and muscular atrophy are also present.

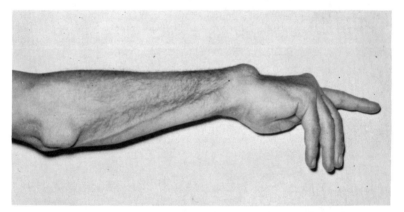

Figure 37.   Dorsal dislocation of the ulna with resultant rupture of extensor tendons of fourth (ring) and fifth (little) fingers of the right hand of a patient with rheumatoid arthritis.

tion of the distal end of the ulna (Fig. 36). Subluxation of the ulna causes abnormal pressure on the extensor communis digitorum tendons, especially those of the fourth and fifth digits, and may result in rupture of these tendons (Fig. 37). Helpful information can be obtained by recognizing any abnormal conditions of the skin (for example, pale, clammy, sweaty, red, atrophic, or hidebound, abnormally tight skin), the presence of nodules, scars of previous operation or trauma, cutaneous lesions, and atrophy of muscles proximal or distal to the wrist.

PALPATION

Wrist

Synovitis in the wrist is indicated by swelling or soft-tissue fullness, with or without tenderness and localized warmth, and is detected most reliably by palpation over the dorsum of the wrist. Because of overlying structures, accurate dorsal and volar localization of the margins of the synovial reflection of the wrist may be difficult. True articular swelling (synovitis) of the wrist is often most palpable just distal to the prominence of the ulna and with palm turned down on the dorsolateral aspect of the wrist because the synovial reflection is more extensive in this region than in other regions of the wrist (Fig. 26).

Palpation of the wrist may be accomplished by use of either of two technics:

1. The examiner faces the patient and supports the patient's hand with his fingers while palpating the wrist firmly with both hands by placing both thumbs on the dorsum of the wrist and both second (index) and third (middle) fingers on the volar aspect of the wrist (Fig. 38). The patient's wrist should be relaxed and in a straight position (0 degrees) with the palm turned down. The palpating thumb is moved above and the palpating fingers below and from side to side over the depressed areas which lie over the region of the joint space just distal to the bony prominences of the radius and ulna. In order to palpate the wrist properly, gentle but firm pressure should be applied by the examining thumb and fingers in order to detect adequately the bony and soft-tissue structures.

2. In an alternative method of examining the wrist the physician supports the patient's hand with one hand while the patient's wrist remains relaxed and in a straight position (0 degrees) with the palm turned down. With his other hand the examining physician then palpates the patient's wrist firmly between his thumb and fingers by placing his thumb on the dorsum of the wrist and his second (index) and third (middle) fingers on the volar aspect of the wrist (Fig. 39). The examiner palpates proximal and distal to the depressed areas of the joint space while moving the examining fingers and thumb across the wrist from one side to the other.

The soft-tissue swelling of synovitis in the wrist can be evaluated further by palpating over the radial aspect of the wrist to detect a palpable bulge when the ulnar side of the wrist joint is compressed.

Sometimes compression of a dorsally located cystic swelling will demonstrate its communication with the wrist joint by causing distention of the articular capsule as the fluid in the cystic swelling is pushed

61

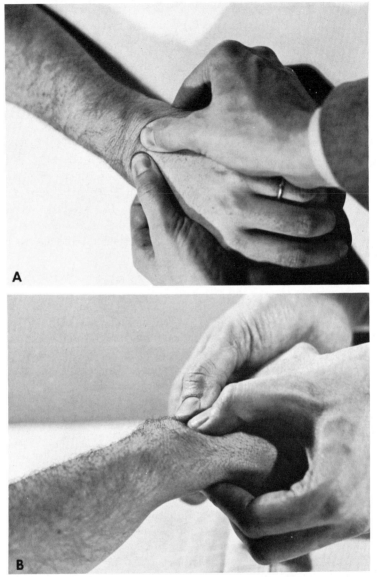

Figure 38. Palpation of the left wrist by using both hands. *A.* Top view. *B.* Side view. The wrist is being palpated firmly (note blanched nails of examiner's thumbs) by both thumbs and second (index) fingers. The other fingers serve to support and position the patient's hand as partially shown in *B.* See text for details.

back temporarily into the wrist joint cavity. If the cyst has resulted from an outpouching of a tendon sheath which does not communicate with the wrist joint, pressure over the cyst will cause distention only over the anatomic distribution of the involved tendon sheath. The close anatomic relationship between the tendon sheaths and the wrist joint often makes it difficult to differentiate localized tenosynovitis from articular synovitis at the level of the wrist. Swelling and tenderness localized to the region of the radial styloid process may result from stenosing tenosynovitis (de Quervain's tenosynovitis) in this area. Additional information also can be obtained by palpating the wrist for nodules on bones or tendons, and for changes in skin temperature.

Palm of Hand and Carpal Joints

After examining the wrist, the examiner may move his fingers distally to palpate the palm and carpal joints. With the examining fingers in the patient's palm and the examining thumbs located on the dorsal aspect of the patient's hand, the physician uses pinching motions in palpating the carpal bones and joints for the presence and localization of swelling, tenderness, and crepitation. Swelling and tenderness in the joints of the carpal bones are often caused by either a mechanical injury or a specific infectious process if they occur without involvement of other joints of the hand or wrist. The localization of involved carpal joints is often difficult by physical examination, and the examiner may need to rely on x-ray changes for precise localization in this area.

Tenosynovitis; Trigger Finger. When the patient's palm is lightly palpated by the examiner while the patient's fingers are slowly and actively flexed and extended, the fine crepitation and thickening indicative of tenosynovitis may be felt. It is helpful for the examiner to place only one of his fingers across the palmar aspect of the metacarpal heads to avoid affecting the patient's ability to make a fist. The patient then actively flexes the metacarpophalangeal joints as far as possible before flexing the proximal and distal interphalangeal joints; this procedure produces a maximal excursion of the flexor tendons and enables the examiner to palpate for crepitation while the tendons move throughout their range of motion. "Rice bodies" or fibrin clumps which give a feeling described as that of "lead shot in a leather bag" may be found by palpation in the presence of some types of chronic tenosynovitis. Sometimes localized cystic outpouchings of the tendon synovial sheaths may be palpated in the palm.

Palpation of the palmar aspect of the hand may reveal nodular enlargement of one or more of the flexor tendons; this almost always occurs at the level of the metacarpal head where a reinforcement or thickening of the deep fascia forms a proximal annular ligament in the sheath of the flexor tendon; this area of thickening is referred to as the "proximal pulley." A finger in which a nodular enlargement of the tendon has developed may become temporarily or even persistently locked in the position of flexion or extension when the tendon is unable to move normally because of a nodular enlargement of the tendon or stenosis of the tendon sheath or both at the level of the

63

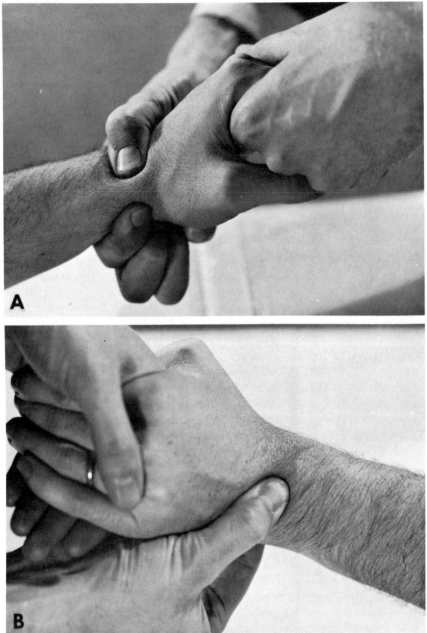

Figure 39.   Palpation of the left wrist using one hand. The examiner's left hand is supporting the patient's hand and wrist in slight dorsiflexion while the examiner's right thumb and second (index) finger are used in pinching motions to examine the joint. A. Palpation of radial aspect of the joint. B. Palpation of mid-portion. C. Palpation of ulnar aspect of the wrist. The examiner palpates above and below the depressed area of the joint space while moving the examining thumb and fingers across the wrist from one side to the other. The blanched nail of the palpating thumb indicates that firm but gentle pressure is applied.

64

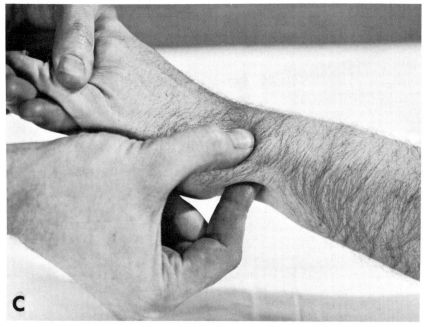

Figure 39. (Continued)

proximal pulley. When additional force is applied and the finger can be moved beyond its fixed position, the nodular enlargement may be pulled through the constricted area, suddenly releasing or snapping the finger into the limit of the range of either extension or flexion, whichever was restricted previously. A click or snap may be felt (and sometimes heard) as the nodular enlargement of the tendon is actively moved past the area of constriction in the tendon sheath. This condition is known as a "trigger" or "snapping" digit. Locking usually occurs when the affected finger is in flexion. Although the flexors of the fingers and thumb are stronger than the extensors, the absence of a tendon sheath on the extensor tendons and the presence of a tendon sheath on the flexor tendons, which may become inflamed, thickened, or stenosed, are probably more significant factors than the comparative strength of the tendons. A trigger or snapping digit involves the first (thumb) and fourth (ring) fingers most frequently but may involve any finger. In patients with rheumatoid arthritis the third (middle) and fourth (ring) fingers are involved more often than the other digits.

Palmar Fascia.   This should be palpated for the presence of fibrous bands and nodules which are to be differentiated from nodular enlargements of flexor tendons. Such palmar nodules are found most often near the distal palmar crease of the fourth digit, but they also may involve the region of the palm near the fifth and third digits.

65

The skin is often irregularly attached over the involved area (Dupuytren's contracture) (Fig. 34).

Special tests for specific conditions will be considered later in this chapter.

MOVEMENT AND RANGE OF MOTION

Movements of the wrist include palmar flexion (flexion), dorsiflexion (extension), radial deviation, and ulnar deviation. A combination of these movements allows circumduction of the wrist. These movements require varying degrees of motion at both the radiocarpal and the midcarpal joints. Limited flexion and extension and slight rotation are permitted in the midcarpal joint. Pronation and supination of the hand and forearm occur primarily at the proximal and distal radio-ulnar articulations.

The carpometacarpal joints move very little with the exception of the carpometacarpal joint of the thumb which possesses the movements of a ball-and-socket joint (flexion, extension, adduction, abduction, and medial and lateral rotation), and which is set at an angle so that flexion and abduction bring the thumb into apposition with the fingers.

The range of wrist motion varies considerably among different individuals and is best evaluated when the examiner grasps the distal end of the patient's forearm proximal to the wrist and allows the patient to demonstrate range of motion actively. Comparisons of wrist motion in the two wrists should be made with both wrists and hands in the same position. It is preferable to examine motion of the wrist with the patient's hand and forearm in pronation since supination and pronation of the hand and forearm influence motion.

Measurements of range of motion in the wrist should start with the wrist and hand in a straight position in relation to the forearm (0 degrees). The wrist usually can be dorsiflexed about 70 degrees and palmar flexed about 80 to 90 degrees from the straight position (Fig. 40). Ulnar deviation averages about 50 to 60 degrees from the straight position and exceeds radial deviation which averages about 20 degrees. Loss of, or limited, dorsiflexion is the most common and important functional impairment of wrist motion.

SPECIAL TESTS FOR INVOLVEMENT OF STRUCTURES
NEAR THE WRIST

Carpometacarpal Joint of the First Digit

The carpometacarpal joint of the thumb is a relatively common site for the changes of degenerative joint disease and sometimes bony

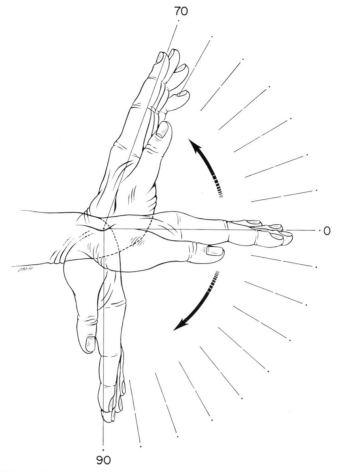

Figure 40.   Range of normal flexion and extension of the wrist.

spurs and crepitation may be felt at the base of the thumb when this joint is involved. Tenderness and swelling or both at the base of the thumb (carpometacarpal joint) should be differentiated from that resulting from involvement of the wrist. The carpometacarpal joint of the thumb can be further evaluated by the following two maneuvers:

1. While the muscles of the patient's thumb are relaxed to avoid symptoms due to muscle spasm or tender muscle attachments, the examiner grasps the thumb near the metacarpophalangeal joint and firmly pushes the thumb inward toward the carpometacarpal joint. This maneuver often produces pain in the region of the carpometacarpal joint if disease of this joint is present.

2. Crepitation of the carpometacarpal joint of the thumb is best palpated at the base of the thumb with the fingers of one of the examiner's hands, while the fingers of the examiner's other hand grasp

67

the patient's thumb in the region of the proximal phalanx and move the patient's thumb in a clockwise rotation.

Stenosing Tenosynovitis at the Radial Styloid Process
(de Quervain's Tenosynovitis)

This condition characteristically involves both the long abductor and short extensor tendons of the thumb (de Quervain's tenosynovitis; Fig. 29). Tenderness near the radial styloid process can be localized further by having the patient place his thumb in the palm of his hand and flex his fingers over the thumb. The patient's hand should be held loosely in this position. If there is no accentuation of the pain or tenderness with the thumb in this position, the examiner grasps the patient's hand and moves the patient's wrist into ulnar deviation cautiously. This maneuver may cause severe pain over the radial styloid process when the test is positive because of the extra tension on the long abductor tendon of the thumb and should be performed with caution when stenosing tenosynovitis is suspected. Comparison with the same maneuver on the opposite side helps one evaluate the patient's reactions.

Compression of the Median Nerve in the Carpal Tunnel
(Carpal Tunnel Syndrome)

This syndrome usually is caused by thickening of the synovial membrane about the flexor tendons. The presence of tenosynovitis often can be observed on inspection when the flexor aspect of the wrist is tangential to the examiner's eyes or can be felt on palpation.

When the wrist is maintained in acute palmar flexion for 60 seconds, numbness and paresthesia often occur in the hand and fingers over the distribution of the median nerve, especially on the palmar surface of the first three digits and a portion of the fourth digit (Phalen's sign). These symptoms are relieved within a few minutes after the wrist assumes a straight position. Sometimes acute extension of the wrist will produce similar symptoms and also should be tried when acute palmar flexion of the wrist does not aggravate median nerve compression. Symptoms also can be produced by placing a blood pressure cuff on the upper arm and inflating it above the level of systolic blood pressure for 3 to 5 minutes. Percussion of the volar aspect of the wrist over the median nerve may be performed to determine whether a tingling or prickling sensation results in the hand over the distribution of the median nerve. The tingling or prickling, when present, suggests compression of the median nerve (Tinel's sign), but it also can occur in individuals without true compression of the median nerve. Decreased sweating on the flexor surface of the digits supplied by the median nerve can be detected in some patients with carpal tunnel syndrome.

Since the flexor pollicis longus, the abductor pollicis brevis, and the opponens pollicis muscles are supplied by the median nerve, they are often weakened when the median nerve is chronically compressed. These muscles, therefore, should be tested when the carpal tunnel syndrome is suspected (see p. 53). Atrophy of the thenar muscles may occur with prolonged median nerve compression (Fig. 35) and is detected by tests described in Chapter 8 (p. 97). Confirmation of weakness and atrophy due to median nerve compression is obtained by electromyographic measurement of the conduction time of the median nerve.

Suggested Reading for Additional Information

1. Byrne, J. J.: The Hand: Its Anatomy and Diseases. Springfield, Illinois, Charles C Thomas, Publisher, 1959, 384 pp.
2. Lampe, E. W.: Surgical Anatomy of the Hand. Ciba Clin. Symposia 9:3–46 (Jan.–Feb.) 1957.
3. Marble, H. C.: The Hand: A Manual and Atlas for the General Surgeon. Philadelphia, W. B. Saunders Company, 1960, 1207 pp.
4. Bunnell, Sterling: Surgery of the Hand. Ed. 3, Philadelphia, J. B. Lippincott Company, 1956, 1079 pp.
5. Steindler, Arthur: Arthritic Deformities of the Wrist and Fingers. J. Bone & Joint Surg. 33-A:849–862, 1951.
6. Flatt, A. E.: The Care of the Rheumatoid Hand. St. Louis, C. V. Mosby Company, 1963, 222 pp.
7. Lipscomb, P. R.: Tenosynovitis of the Hand and the Wrist: Carpal Tunnel Syndrome, de Quervain's Disease, Trigger Digit. Clin. Orthopaedics 13:164–181, 1959.
8. Brewerton, D. A.: Hand Deformities in Rheumatoid Disease. Ann. Rheumat. Dis. 16:183–197 (June) 1957.
9. Vaughan-Jackson, O. J.: Rheumatoid Hand Deformities Considered in the Light of Tendon Imbalances. J. Bone & Joint Surg. 44-B:764–775, 1962.
10. Backdahl, M.: The Caput Ulnae Syndrome in Rheumatoid Arthritis: A Study of the Morphology, Abnormal Anatomy and Clinical Picture. Acta rheumat. scandinav. Suppl. 5, 1963, pp. 1–75.
11. American Academy of Orthopaedic Surgeons: Measuring and Recording of Joint Motion. Everett, Massachusetts, Glenwood Press, 1963, 91 pp.

CHAPTER EIGHT

METACARPOPHALANGEAL, PROXIMAL AND DISTAL INTERPHALANGEAL JOINTS

ESSENTIAL ANATOMY

> Joints, Ligaments, and Tendons
> > *Metacarpophalangeal joints*
> > *Proximal and distal interphalangeal joints*
> Articular Capsule and Synovial Membrane

INSPECTION

PALPATION

> Metacarpophalangeal Joints
> Proximal Interphalangeal Joints
> Distal Interphalangeal Joints

MOVEMENT AND RANGE OF MOTION OF THE DIGITS, INCLUDING METACARPOPHALAN-GEAL, PROXIMAL INTERPHALANGEAL AND DISTAL INTERPHALANGEAL JOINTS

> Range of Motion
> Testing for Muscle Strength

ESSENTIAL ANATOMY

Joints, Ligaments, and Tendons

Metacarpophalangeal Joints.   These joints (which are hinge joints) have dense fibrous or fibrocartilaginous ligaments over the palmar surface (known as the volar plate) and are reinforced by collateral ligaments on each side. These collateral ligaments which become

70

tight in flexion and loose in extension prevent lateral motion of the digit distal to the metacarpophalangeal joint when it is flexed. An extensor tendon crosses the dorsum of each joint and strengthens the thin articular capsule in this region. When the extensor tendon of the digit reaches the distal end of the metacarpal head, it is joined by fibers of the interossei and lumbricales, and thus expands over the entire dorsum of the metacarpophalangeal joint and onto the dorsum of the adjacent phalanx. This expansion of the extensor mechanism is known as the extensor hood. Opposite the metacarpophalangeal joint each extensor tendon is bound by fasciculi to the collateral ligaments. (The anatomy of the flexor tendons of the hand is discussed in Chapter 7, p. 53.)

Proximal and Distal Interphalangeal Joints. These are similar anatomically. They are true hinge joints whose movements are restricted to flexion and extension. The ligaments of the interphalangeal joints resemble those of the metacarpophalangeal joints. Each interphalangeal joint has a thin dorsal capsular ligament strengthened by expansion of the extensor tendon, a dense palmar ligament (volar plate), and collateral ligaments which strengthen each side of the joint. Opposite the proximal interphalangeal joint the extensor tendon divides into three slips: one intermediate and two collateral. The intermediate slip is inserted into the base of the second phalanx, and the two collateral slips extend along the sides of the second phalanx to unite and insert into the dorsal surface of the terminal phalanx. The palmar and collateral ligaments normally help prevent hyperextension of the proximal and distal interphalangeal joints.

Articular Capsule and Synovial Membrane

When the fingers are flexed, the heads of the metacarpal bones form the rounded prominences of the knuckles with the metacarpophalangeal joint spaces lying about 1 cm. distal to the apices of these prominences (Fig. 41). The distal part of the articular capsule and the synovial membrane which lines the inner surface of the capsule are both attached firmly to the base of the proximal phalanx and the metacarpal head, but the articular capsule is loose over the metacarpal head (Figs. 26 and 27). Figure 26 shows the relationship of the dorsal aspect of the joint space, the synovial membrane, and the articular capsule to adjacent and overlying structures. The skin on the palmar surface of the hand is relatively thick and covers a fat pad between it and the metacarpophalangeal joint; this makes palpation of the palmar surface of the joint space and articular capsule more difficult and less satisfactory than palpation of the dorsolateral surfaces (Fig. 27).

The distribution of the articular capsule and synovial membrane of the proximal and distal interphalangeal joints is similar to that of

71

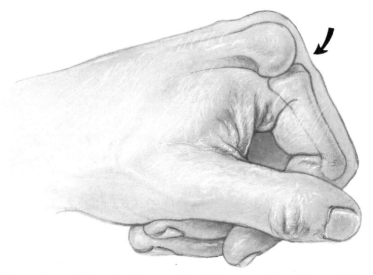

Figure 41.   Schematic diagram of medial aspect of hand. Arrow indicates that the metacarpophalangeal joint space lies distal to the prominence of the knuckle when the proximal phalanx is flexed on the metacarpophalangeal joint.

the metacarpophalangeal joint. Both the synovial membrane and the articular capsule of the interphalangeal joints are firmly attached distally to the base of the more distal phalanx forming the joint and firmly, but more extensively, to the phalanx forming the proximal portion of the joint (Fig. 27).

INSPECTION (FIGS. 42 THROUGH 61)

Swelling of the metacarpophalangeal and interphalangeal joints may result from articular or periarticular causes. The loss of normal knuckle wrinkles is indicative of soft-tissue swelling and suggests synovitis of the involved joints if the swelling is restricted to the distribution of the synovial membrane and articular capsule. Synovial swelling (Figs. 42 and 45) produces symmetrical enlargement of the joint, whereas extra-articular swelling (Figs. 44 and 59) may be diffuse and is often asymmetrical, involving one side of the joint but not the other. This differentiation is exemplified by comparison of Figures 42 and 44; Figure 42 shows synovitis in the metacarpophalangeal joints while Figure 44 shows diffuse edema on the dorsum of the hands and in the region of the metacarpophalangeal joints.

Synovial distention or thickening of a metacarpophalangeal joint may produce stretching and eventual relaxation of the articular capsule and ligaments. This combined with muscle imbalance and the force

72

of gravity may cause the extensor tendon of the digit to slip off the metacarpal head on the ulnar side of the joint. The abnormal pull of the tendon resulting from this displacement may contribute significantly to the development of an ulnar deviation or "drift" of the fingers (Figs. 42, 48 and 49). However, the exact mechanism of the ulnar deviation of the fingers is not well understood as yet, and it is probable that ulnar deviation results from multiple factors which may vary in different instances. When ulnar deviation of the fingers occurs, subluxation of the proximal phalanx or phalanges of the fingers at the metacarpophalangeal joint or joints often is associated.

Hyperextension of the proximal interphalangeal joints results when the interossei or the lateral expansion of the extensor mechanism becomes thickened and shortened or the extensor tendon is pushed dorsally by the distended joint capsule. In the hyperextended position, flexion of the interphalangeal joints is difficult for the patient to initiate. Hyperextension of the proximal interphalangeal joint is often associated with partial flexion of the distal interphalangeal joint due to tightening of the flexor tendon to the terminal phalanx.

The term "swan-neck deformity" is used to describe the appearance of a finger resulting from contracture of the interossei and flexor muscles or tendons that produces a flexion contracture of the metacarpophalangeal joint, sequential hyperextension of the proximal interphalangeal joint, and flexion of the distal interphalangeal joint (Fig. 46). The term "swan-neck deformity" was suggested because the contracture resembles the curved shape of a swan's neck. A similar deformity characterized by flexion of the metacarpophalangeal joint and hyperextension of the interphalangeal joint may occur in the thumb. Such contractures often are accompanied by ulnar drift of the fingers.

When a swan-neck deformity is present, the patient is unable to flex the proximal interphalangeal joint while the metacarpophalangeal joint of the affected digit (or digits) is held in extension. When it is noted that the proximal interphalangeal joints cannot be actively flexed in this position, the examiner should passively flex all three of the joints of the digit to determine whether the limitation of interphalangeal flexion results from the swan-neck deformity, from destructive disease of the joint, or from involvement of the extensor tendons.

In the normal hand there is a balance between the pull exerted by the long flexors, the long extensors, and the intrinsic muscles. When the intrinsic muscles and their tendons exert an "overpull," the hand develops "intrinsic-plus" contractures such as the "swan-neck" deformity just described. If the intrinsic muscles are paralyzed by loss of innervation from both the median and ulnar nerves, the hand assumes an "intrinsic-minus" position usually referred to as a paralytic or "claw" hand. A claw hand is characterized by hyperextension of the meta-

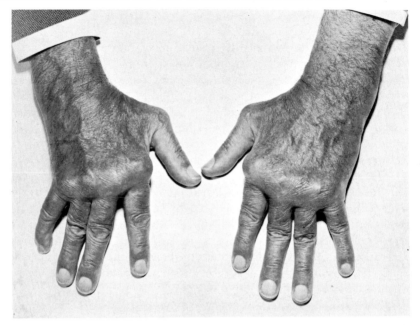

Figure 42. Characteristic soft-tissue swelling (synovitis, grade 2) and flexion contractures of the metacarpophalangeal joints and hyperextension of proximal interphalangeal joints of second to fifth digits, inclusive, in a patient with advanced rheumatoid arthritis. Ulnar deviation of the fingers is especially evident in patient's right hand. Muscular atrophy of hands and synovitis of wrists are also present.

carpophalangeal joints, flexion of the proximal and distal interphalangeal joints, flattening or loss of the metacarpal arch, and adduction and external rotation of the thumb.

The term "boutonnière deformity" is used to describe flexion of the proximal interphalangeal joint accompanied by compensatory hyperextension of the distal interphalangeal joint of the same digit (Fig. 46). This relatively common deformity results from detachment of the central slip of the extensor tendon of the proximal interphalangeal joint from the base of the middle phalanx which thus allows dislocation of the lateral bands in a palmar direction. When the dislocated lateral bands cross the fulcrum of the joint, they act as flexors, instead of extensors, of the joint. As a result of this distortion, the proximal and distal phalanges of the joint are pushed between the two dislocated lateral bands. The anatomic appearance is that of a knuckle being pushed through a buttonhole, hence the derivation of the term "boutonnière deformity."

Helpful information is obtained from recognition of abnormalities of the terminal digits, including bony, soft-tissue, and nail changes. Bony changes may be evident as osteophytic articular nodules. When

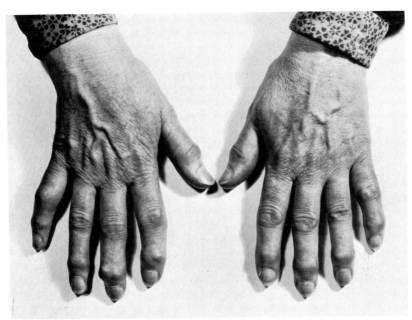

Figure 43.   Degenerative joint disease (osteoarthritis) of both hands. Osteoarthritic enlargement of the distal interphalangeal joints (Heberden's nodes) and the proximal interphalangeal joints (Bouchard's nodes) is present. The metacarpophalangeal joints are not affected.

these occur on the distal interphalangeal joints, they are described as Heberden's nodes and when on the proximal interphalangeal joints as Bouchard's nodes; similar nodules result from trauma, infection or chronic inflammation. Telescopic shortening of the digits produced by resorption of the ends of the phalanges is associated with wrinkling of the skin over the involved joints (opera-glass hand or "main en lorgnette").

Soft-tissue changes include synovial cysts on the dorsolateral aspects of the joints (Fig. 52), thickening of the fibrous capsule which produces an extra-articular swelling on the dorsum of the proximal interphalangeal joints ("dorsal knuckle pads"; Fig 61), and clubbing of the terminal phalanges (Fig. 56). The latter is sometimes associated with hypertrophic pulmonary osteoarthropathy. Other changes include the presence of soft-tissue nodules or urate tophi (Fig. 53). Nail changes include pitting, ridging, thickening, discoloration (Fig. 55) or watch-crystal rounding (Fig. 56). The latter may be associated with clubbing of the terminal phalanx. Changes in the skin include pallor, rubor, edema, atrophy, ulcers, and hidebound tightening. Figures 42 through 61 give examples of types of conditions visible on inspection.

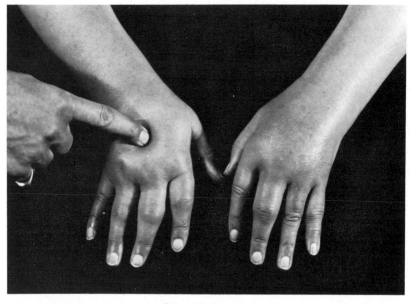

Figure 44.   Massive diffuse edema of both hands associated with but obscuring synovitis of the wrists and metacarpophalangeal joints. The swelling in the proximal interphalangeal joints, especially evident in the third finger of each hand, is in the distribution of the synovial membrane and can be differentiated on palpation from the edema extending into the area of the proximal phalanx from the dorsum of the hand. Patient had rheumatoid arthritis.

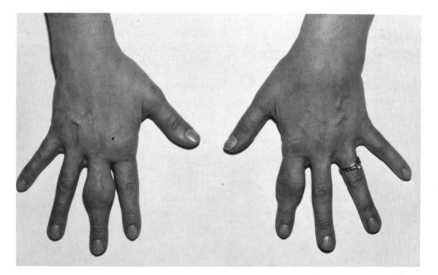

Figure 45.   Marked fusiform swelling of proximal interphalangeal joints of third digit in right hand (synovitis, grade 4) and second digit in left hand (synovitis, grade 3) in patient with rheumatoid arthritis. Fusiform swelling of the proximal interphalangeal joints commonly occurs in rheumatoid arthritis, but it is more characteristically symmetrical than is the asymmetrical involvement of the fingers shown here.

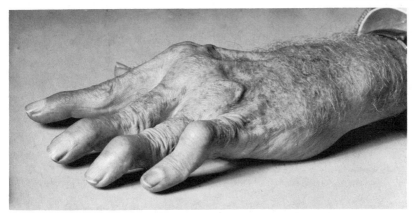

Figure 46.   Flexion of the metacarpophalangeal joints, hyperextension of the proximal interphalangeal joints and flexion of distal interphalangeal joints in the second, third, and fourth digits in patient with rheumatoid arthritis ("intrinsic" plus or "swan-neck" deformity). In the fifth digit the proximal interphalangeal joint is flexed and the distal interphalangeal joint is hyperextended (boutonnière deformity).

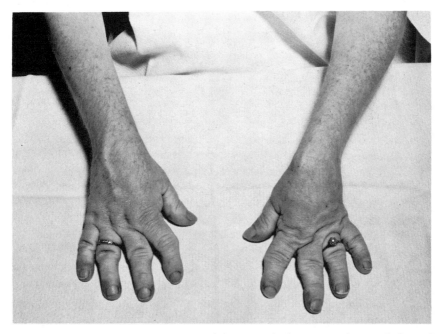

Figure 47.   Hyperextension deformity of the proximal interphalangeal joints of patient whose rheumatoid arthritis had a juvenile onset and was associated with stunting of growth. Arthropathic resorption of phalanges and articulations resulted in wrinkling and redundancy of the skin of the digits and hypermobility of metacarpophalangeal and proximal interphalangeal joints. This photograph also shows synovial swelling of both wrists. The patient also had limited motion of these joints.

77

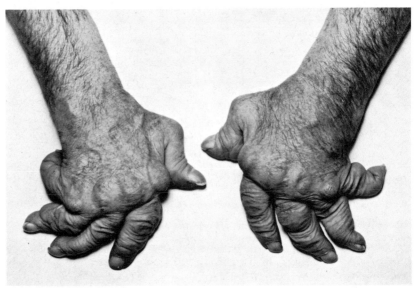

Figure 48.   Severe deformities of both hands in patient with advanced rheumatoid arthritis. There is chronic synovitis and subluxation of metacarpophalangeal joints, marked ulnar deviation of fingers, shortening of digits and wrinkling of skin over damaged joints, producing the opera-glass hand or "la main en lorgnette."

PALPATION

Metacarpophalangeal Joints

The metacarpophalangeal joint is palpated for evidence of synovial thickening or distention, tenderness, and warmth in three locations: in the region of the joint space, over the metacarpal head, and in the groove between adjacent metacarpal heads. Normally the synovial membrane cannot be palpated in the region of the joint space, but in the presence of synovial thickening the bony margins of the joint space are obscured by swelling. The joint space is felt most easily with the proximal phalanx flexed about 20 to 30 degrees on the metacarpophalangeal joint and about 1 cm. distal to the apex of the knuckles (Fig. 41). It is palpated best over the dorsolateral aspects of the joint on each side of the extensor tendon (Fig. 62).

The extensor tendon of the digit can be delineated easily in the midline as it crosses the dorsum of the joint, but adequate examination of the portion of the joint directly beneath this structure is not possible under normal conditions. Distention of the synovial membrane and articular capsule, however, may cause stretching and eventual relaxation of the articular capsule and ligaments so that the extensor tendon of the digit is allowed to slip off the prominence of the metacarpal

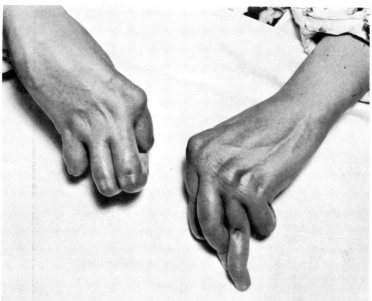

Figure 49. Another type of severe deformity of the fingers in patient with rheumatoid arthritis. The right wrist is swollen and ankylosed in mild flexion. The metacarpophalangeal joints of the third, fourth, and fifth digits on the right are hyperextended and there are flexion contractures of the proximal interphalangeal joints of these digits. The metacarpophalangeal joints of the left hand are flexed, the proximal interphalangeal joints of the second and fourth digits are hyperextended, and the distal interphalangeal joints in the same digits are flexed (swan-neck deformity). The proximal interphalangeal joints of the left third and fifth digits are flexed, the distal interphalangeal joint of the left third digit is hyperextended, and that of the fifth digit is flexed but not fully visualized in this photograph. Ulnar deviation is present in both hands but is more marked on the left.

head. When this occurs, the tendon can be palpated on the ulnar side of the metacarpal head in the longitudinal groove between adjacent metacarpal heads, and then the exposed joint space can be palpated easily over the dorsal aspect of the joint.

The region of the joint space is palpated with the joint partially flexed, and then the metacarpal head and joint space also are palpated with the joint extended. The finger of the metacarpophalangeal joint being examined is held in extension by the examiner's fingers during the examination, as this relaxes the articular capsule and enables the examiner to feel synovial thickening more easily (Fig. 63). Extension of the metacarpophalangeal joint accentuates any soft-tissue swelling of synovitis but also may cause distention of periarticular tissues which needs to be differentiated from synovial swelling.

The region over the metacarpal head and the longitudinal groove between adjacent metacarpal heads also are palpated for evidence of synovial thickening or distention. Normally the synovial membrane can-

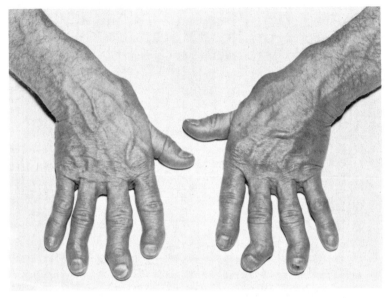

Figure 50.   Deviation of the distal phalanx at the distal interphalangeal joint in the second, third, and fourth digits of the right hand and in the third and fourth digits of the left hand in patient with degenerative joint disease (osteoarthritis). Heberden's nodes are seen at the distal interphalangeal joints, and some bony enlargement is present in the proximal interphalangeal joints and there is a bony prominence of the carpometacarpal joint at the base of each thumb.

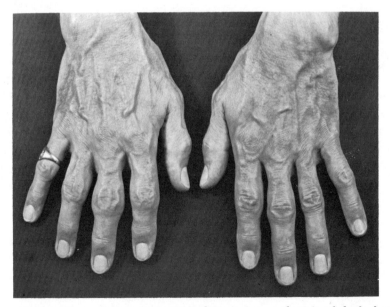

Figure 51.   Degenerative joint disease (osteoarthritis) of both hands. Bony enlargement of proximal interphalangeal joints, Heberden's nodes in distal interphalangeal joints, and characteristic sparing of the metacarpophalangeal joints should be noted.

80

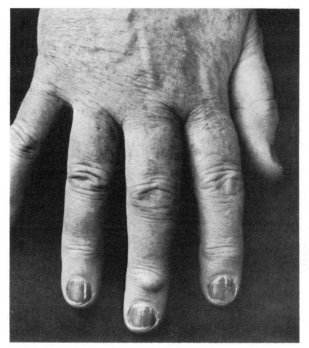

Figure 52. Synovial cyst from distal interphalangeal joint of third digit of patient with Heberden's nodes.

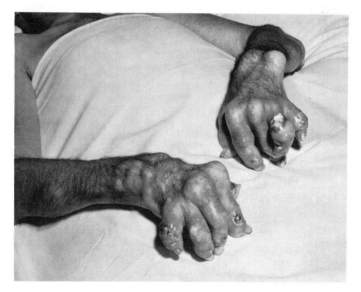

Figure 53. Multiple tophi in forearms, wrists, and hands with ulceration and drainage of urates from tophi in several proximal and distal interphalangeal joints of patient with severe chronic gouty arthritis.

81

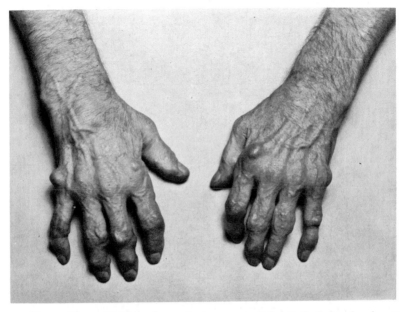

Figure 54.   Multiple firm subcutaneous nodules in both hands of patient with rheumatoid arthritis.

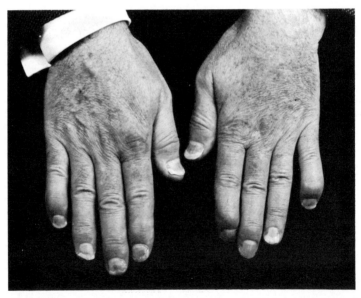

Figure 55.   Swelling and flexion of several distal interphalangeal joints and pitting, discoloration, and elevation of terminal portion of nails in patient with psoriatic arthritis.

82

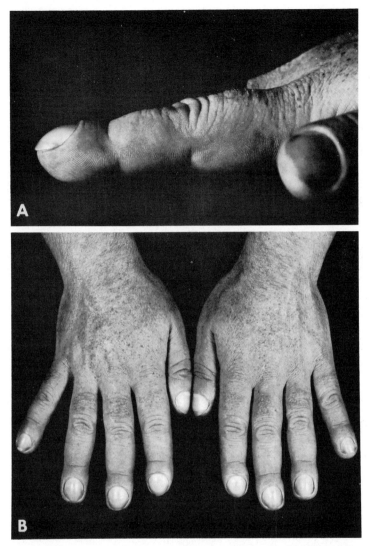

Figure 56.   Clubbing of distal interphalangeal joints and rounding of the nails in a patient with hypertrophic osteoarthropathy. *A.* Close up, side view of index finger. *B.* Dorsal aspect of both hands.

not be palpated in this groove, but in the presence of synovial thickening or distention, the groove on both sides of the involved joint and the normal hard bony landmarks of the metacarpal heads and the joint spaces are obliterated. Synovial thickening can be evaluated more completely by rolling the palpating thumb and finger or both thumbs over the dorsolateral aspects of the metacarpal heads (Fig. 64). Interpretation of the examination would be facilitated by again referring to the anatomy and the attachments of the synovial membrane described

83

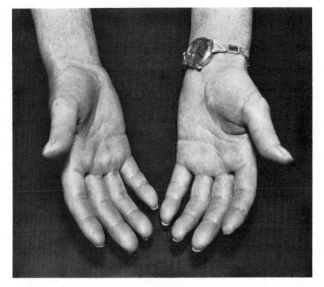

Figure 57.   Diffuse puffiness of fingers but no atrophy or contractures in patient with csleroderma and early acrosclerosis.

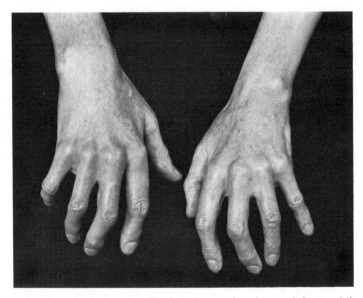

Figure 58.   Tight, shiny, hidebound, atrophic skin, and flexion deformities at the proximal interphalangeal joints in a stage of scleroderma with acrosclerosis more advanced than in Figure 57.

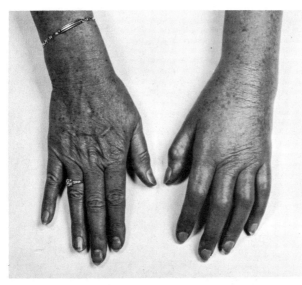

Figure 59. Diffuse edema and swelling in left hand (associated with limitation of left shoulder) in early stage of shoulder-hand syndrome.

Figure 60. Palmar fascial atrophy and contractures and flexion deformities of fingers of both hands in the late (residual) stage of bilateral shoulder-hand syndrome.

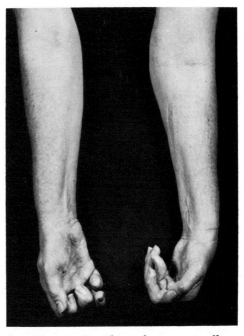

in the section on "Anatomy" and in Figure 41. The soft-tissue swelling of synovitis is symmetrical in relation to the involved joint and may be associated with warmth and tenderness. If soft-tissue swelling is present only on one side of a metacarpal head, it most likely lies outside the articular capsule and is not due to an intra-articular reaction.

85

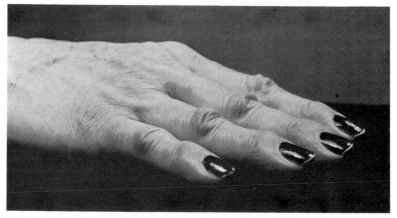

Figure 61.   Thickening and elevation of skin and subcutaneous tissues on dorsal aspect of proximal interphalangeal joints without evidence of arthritis. This condition is known as "dorsal knuckle pads."

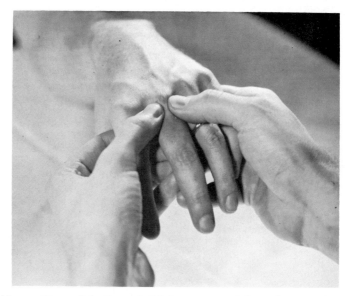

Figure 62.   Palpation of third metacarpophalangeal joint of left hand. Examiner's thumbs are palpating dorsal aspect of joint while forefingers (not seen in this photograph) are palpating volar aspect of metacarpal head. The joint being examined is held in a relaxed position of partial flexion. The examiner's remaining fingers support the patient's hand. The other metacarpophalangeal joints are similarly examined. Compare with Figure 41 showing the position of joint relative to the prominence of the knuckle.

To palpate the metacarpophalangeal joint, the patient's hand should be relaxed and in as comfortable a position as possible with the palm turned down and the wrist in pronation. Each joint is examined separately by grasping the joint firmly between both of the examiner's thumbs which are placed on the dorsum of the joint and both index

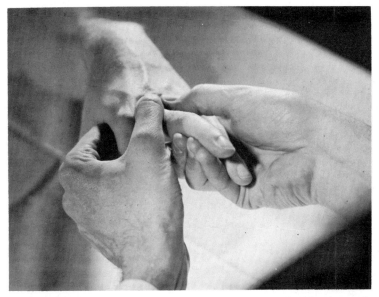

Figure 63. Alternate position for palpation over dorsal aspect of meta-carpophalangeal joints. The palpating thumbs are proximal to the level of the joint line (see Fig. 42). The joint is examined in a position midway between hyper-extension and dorsiflexion or in slight hyperextension as shown here. The position and function of the examiner's digits are similar to those shown and described in Figure 62.

fingers which are placed on the palmar aspect of the joint while the examiner's remaining fingers support the patient's head (Fig. 62). In an alternative method, the examiner palpates the dorsal aspect of the joint between the thumb and index finger of one hand while his other hand supports the patient's hand. With either method, examination of the metacarpophalangeal joint should include palpation of the joint space, the metacarpal head and the longitudinal groove between ad-jacent metacarpal heads for evidence of synovial thickening or distention with the joint flexed and also with the joint extended (Figs. 62, 63 and 64).

The examiner's index fingers, when placed on the palmar surface of the metacarpal head, should feel for tenderness and fullness while the joint is compressed between the examiner's thumbs on the dorsal surface and the index fingers. Subluxation of the proximal phalanx on the metacarpal head may occur toward the palmar aspect of the hand; when this happens, the bony landmarks of the adjacent phalanx are more prominent than they are normally.

If an "intrinsic plus" muscle contracture is present, the meta-carpophalangeal joint cannot be extended fully, and when full extension is attempted passively, the proximal interphalangeal joint goes into hyper-extension and the distal interphalangeal joint into flexion, producing

87

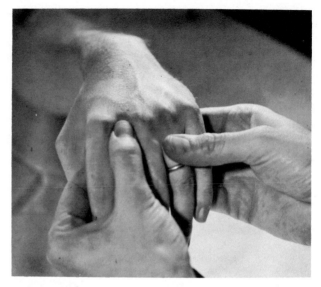

Figure 64.   Palpation in groove between adjacent metacarpal heads of left hand for evidence of synovitis. The left thumb of the examiner is palpating deeply. It is alternatively turned to feel each adjacent metacarpal head and joint. The examiner's right hand and the digits of the left hand not being used in palpation are used to support the patient's hand. The joint being examined is slightly flexed. See text for details.

the swan-neck deformity of the digit. If this condition is accompanied by ulnar drift of the fingers, the contractures are accentuated when the examiner passively moves the digit toward the radial side of the hand to bring the finger back to its realigned straight position in relationship to its metacarpal.

Proximal Interphalangeal Joint

In palpation of the proximal interphalangeal joint, the soft-tissue swelling of knuckle pads on the dorsal aspect and tenosynovial reactions of flexor tendon sheaths must be distinguished from true synovial reactions involving the joint. Synovial swelling indicates a reaction throughout the synovial membrane; local tenderness, warmth, or redness may or may not be associated. Swelling is most readily palpable on the medial and lateral aspects of the joint and just proximal to the joint space because of the looser and more extensive attachment of the synovial membrane to the proximal phalanx as compared to the middle phalanx and because an expansion of the extensor tendon of the digit covers the dorsum of the proximal interphalangeal joint. The soft-tissue swelling of tenosynovitis usually involves the palmar aspect of the joint and may be associated with tenderness, local warmth, induration, and locking or crepitation when motion of the digit is attempted. Thickening of the skin and subcutaneous tissue over the dorsal aspect of the proximal interphalangeal joints (knuckle pad) appears as localized, superficial nontender swelling without local heat or redness and with a firmer consistency than that of synovial distention and should not be confused with swelling in the distribution of the synovial membrane or joint capsule.

When diffuse swelling of the digits occurs, it extends over the region of the joint as well as between the joints and makes it difficult or impossible to palpate through this swelling to evaluate intra-articular synovial reactions. Palpable bony enlargement of articular margins can be differentiated without difficulty from the "boggy" soft-tissue reaction of synovial swelling.

In palpation of the proximal interphalangeal joint, the examiner supports the patient's hand with one hand while palpating each proximal interphalangeal joint between the thumb and index finger of his other hand placed on each side of the joint being examined (Fig. 65). Additional information concerning swelling and tenderness of the proximal interphalangeal joint may be obtained when the examiner places his

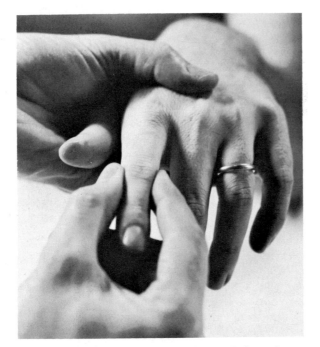

Figure 65. Palpation of the proximal interphalangeal joint of the left second finger. The examiner's left hand is supporting the patient's hand while the examiner's right thumb and forefinger are used to palpate simultaneously and alternately the medial and lateral aspects of the joint. The other proximal interphalangeal joints are examined similarly. See text for details.

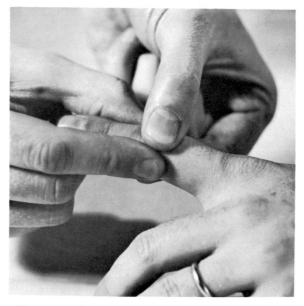

Figure 66. An alternate technic for palpation of synovial distention in proximal interphalangeal joint is illustrated here on the proximal interphalangeal joint of the second finger on the left hand. The joint capsule is first compressed antero-posteriorly between the examiner's left thumb and second finger while the examiner's right thumb (medial) and second finger (lateral) lightly palpate for fluctuant synovial distention. Then the right thumb and finger compress the joint capsule while the left thumb and finger palpate. The firmness with which the joint is examined is illustrated by the blanching of the examiner's nails, but palpation also should be performed gently and lightly.

thumb over the dorsal surface and his index finger over the palmar surface and the thumb and index finger of his other hand over the medial and lateral aspects of the joint, respectively (Fig. 66). Pressure is applied by the digits of the examiner's hands on the dorsal and palmar surfaces to distend maximally the synovial membrane to each side of the joint where it then may be palpated more easily.

Distal Interphalangeal Joint

To palpate each distal interphalangeal joint, the examiner places a thumb and index finger on opposite sides of the joint since articular tenderness, swelling, or local heat is most readily detected on the dorso-medial and dorsolateral aspects of the joint. Hard, and usually non-tender, bony enlargements (Heberden's nodes) are palpated earliest as a ridge over the dorsum of the distal interphalangeal joint but when larger may be more prominently felt medially and laterally. Synovial cysts from joints and tendon sheaths have a cystic consistency which may or may not be compressible and by which they may be recognized;

90

tenderness, local heat, or warmth is usually absent. Synovial cysts of joints develop as an outpouching of the synovial membrane through the articular capsule and are usually located on the dorsal, dorsomedial, or dorsolateral aspect of the joint. Synovial cysts of tendon sheaths usually occur on the palmar or volar aspect of the digit.

The technic of examining the distal interphalangeal joint is exactly the same as that of examining the proximal interphalangeal joint. The examiner, however, should be aware of the marked difference in predilection of the two interphalangeal joints for certain types of disease. Thus Heberden's nodes, clubbing, and psoriatic arthritis characteristically affect the distal interphalangeal joint, and rheumatoid arthritis commonly involves the proximal interphalangeal joint more than the distal interphalangeal joint. Detachment of the extensor tendon from the base of the distal phalanx produces a flexion deformity of the distal phalanx and hyperextension of the middle interphalangeal joint (mallet finger).

MOVEMENT AND RANGE OF MOTION OF THE DIGITS, INCLUDING METACARPOPHALANGEAL, PROXIMAL INTERPHALANGEAL AND DISTAL INTERPHALANGEAL JOINTS

Movement of the digits should be evaluated as a unit, and then the movement of each joint can be evaluated separately. A simple measure of over-all function of the fingers is the ability of the patient to make a complete fist and to extend the fingers fully. Movement of the fingers as a whole thus may be observed by asking the patient to flex and then extend his fingers as far as possible (active motion). The thumb should be sufficiently abducted so that it does not interfere with flexion of the fingers or give a misleading impression of a tight fist when the ability to make a fist is actually impaired. A normal complete fist produced by complete flexion of all the fingers is described as a 100 per cent fist, and a flat hand with no flexion of the fingers would be considered a 0 per cent fist. Examples of approximately 25, 50, and 75 per cent fists are shown in Figure 67. Composite flexion of all of the joints of the fingers can also be determined by measuring the distance from the tips of the flexed fingers to the proximal crease of the palm.

The lack of full extension of the fingers is measured best in degrees of full extension which may be lacking (for example, the fingers may lack 10, 20, or 30 degrees of full extension). After the patient has flexed and extended his fingers actively, the examiner moves each of the metacarpophalangeal joints to its complete flexion and, while holding the fingers in this position, moves each of the proximal interphalangeal joints to complete flexion, and then moves each of the distal

91

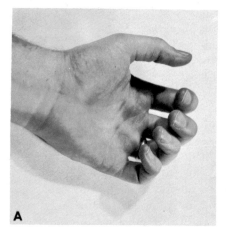

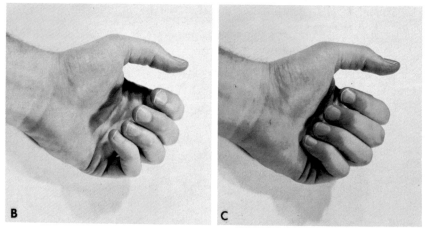

Figure 67. Illustrations of approximate degrees of flexion of the fingers used in making a fist. A. Twenty-five per cent fist. B. Fifty per cent fist. C. Seventy-five per cent fist. A complete fist (not illustrated) would be recorded as 100 per cent fist.

interphalangeal joints to complete flexion. The patient's wrist must be extended slightly, and the hand should remain relaxed during these maneuvers in order to evaluate motion of the fingers adequately and correctly. Muscle weakness or "trigger" digits cause limitation of active motion without impairing the range of passive motion. Subluxation of metacarpophalangeal joints is particularly apparent during active flexion of the metacarpophalangeal joints. When this occurs, the distal bone of the metacarpophalangeal joint (proximal end of the adjacent phalanx) should be supported by pressure of the examiner's finger against the palmar aspect of the patient's phalanx throughout the range of passive movement of the metacarpophalangeal joint in order to reduce the dislocation as much as possible and thereby evaluate more accurately the movement of the joints of the fingers distal to the metacarpo-phalangeal joints.

Range of Motion

In determining range of motion in individual joints, the examiner should note whether each of the digital joints contributes normally to the total range observed. The proximal interphalangeal joints, for example, may flex completely to enable the fingertips to touch or almost touch the distal portion of the palm, but flexion at the metacarpopha-langeal joints may be incomplete. Or the metacarpophalangeal joints may flex well, but the fingers may be unable to touch the proximal portion of the palm because motion at the proximal interphalangeal joints is limited. Such limitation, however, is not necessarily in the joint.

A greater limitation of passive motion as compared to active motion may occur in any joint affected by pain and swelling. Passive movement of the metacarpophalangeal joints is greater than active move-ment in the presence of certain types of stenosing tenosynovitis. Rupture of either flexor or extensor tendons also limits active movement of the fingers to a greater degree than it limits passive motion. When the range of motion is limited and voluntary or active motion equals passive motion, the limitation can be attributed to involvement of the joint, to tightening of the articular capsule and periarticular tissues by distention or fibrosis, or to fixed muscle contractures.

The range of motion in the metacarpophalangeal joints results from flexion-extension or abduction-adduction of the proximal phalanges on the metacarpal heads; a combination of these movements allows circumduction. The collateral ligaments are loose in extension and tight in flexion; thus they produce a firm grasp without lateral motion of the fingers when the metacarpophalangeal joint is flexed. The meta-carpophalangeal joint of the thumb moves more like a hinge joint since its lateral motion is restricted. The proximal and distal interphalangeal joints are true hinge joints whose movement is restricted to flexion and extension in contrast to the range of motion in the metacarpophalangeal joints. Hyperextension normally is prevented by the palmar and col-lateral ligaments. Flexion at the proximal interphalangeal joint is greater than flexion at the distal interphalangeal joint.

To measure the degree of flexion in a joint of any finger, the examiner supports the proximal phalanx while the patient demonstrates range of motion by moving the distal phalanx or phalanges (active motion) or the examiner moves the distal phalanx or phalanges (passive motion). The metacarpophalangeal joints of the fingers flex about 90 to 100 degrees from the normal neutral (0 degree) extended position (Figs. 68 and 69). The metacarpophalangeal joint of the thumb, how-

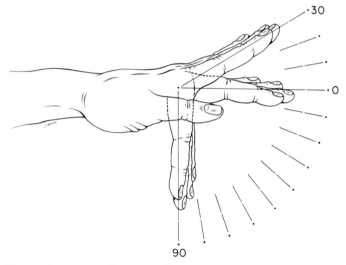

Figure 68. Normal range of flexion and extension in metacarpophalangeal joints of fingers.

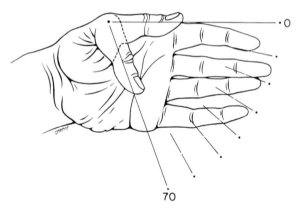

Figure 69. Normal range of flexion in metacarpophalangeal joint of thumb (first digit).

ever, flexes only to about 50 degrees. The proximal interphalangeal joints flex 100 to 120 degrees, and the distal interphalangeal joints flex 45 to 90 degrees also from the neutral (0 degree) extended position (Figs. 70 and 71).

Each metcarpophalangeal joint may hyperextend as much as 30 degrees from the neutral (0 degree) extended position, but some individuals are unable to extend the metacarpophalangeal joint farther than the neutral extended position. The proximal interphalangeal joint rarely hyperextends more than 10 degrees. The distal interphalangeal joint may hyperextend as much as 30 degrees, but there is considerable variation, and some individuals cannot extend either joint farther than the neutral extended position. The interphalangeal joint of the thumb commonly hyperextends about 20 to 35 degrees and flexes to about 80 to 90 degrees (Fig. 72). Each of the fingers is capable of abduction (spreading of the fingers) and adduction (movement of fingers toward the third or middle finger) when the metacarpophalangeal joint is extended. The complete range of abduction-adduction at the metacarpophalangeal joint is approximately 30 to 40 degrees, but the relative contribution of abduction and adduction varies from joint to joint. There is minimal abduction or adduction at the metacarpophalangeal joint of the thumb, and most of this type of motion in the thumb plus

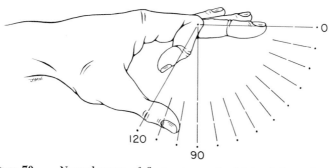

Figure 70.   Normal range of flexion in proximal interphalangeal joint.

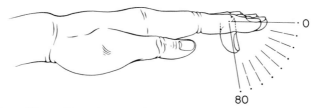

Figure 71.   Normal range of flexion in distal interphalangeal joint.

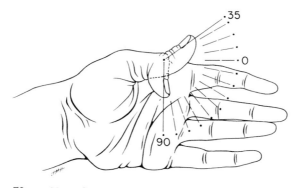

Figure 72.   Normal range of flexion and extension in interphalangeal joint of thumb (first digit).

the motion due to function of the opponens muscle occurs at the carpo-metacarpal articulation. Abduction at the carpometacarpal articulation may be measured parallel to or at a right angle to the plane of the palm and is about 70 degrees in each plane.

Destruction of the joint and laxity of the articular capsule and ligaments produced by synovial swelling may cause instability of finger joints and eventually lead to dislocation and hypermobile, or flail joints Passive and even the active range of motion in a subluxed or dislocated joint can sometimes be tested in the following manner: When the bony structures forming the joint are supported by the examiner in their normal position, the range of motion in the joint may be greater than it is when the joint is subluxed. Considerable improvement in the range of active flexion and extension in a subluxed finger joint when the examiner holds the joint structures in their normal position indicates relatively good potential function of the joint and intact flexor and extensor tendons.

Testing for Muscle Strength

When the patient makes a fist by grasping two or more of the examiner's fingers, a general estimate of muscular strength can be made, but the strength of the individual muscles of the hand needs to be evaluated separately in the presence of any abnormality of the grip or inability to extend the fingers. The interossei muscles are supplied by the ulnar nerve and can be evaluated by testing the strength of the digits in adduction and abduction against resistance. To measure abduction of the patient's extended digit, the examiner applies resistance with his finger to each of the patient's fingers while the patient holds his fingers spread apart. The resistance is directed toward the patient's middle finger. Adduction can be tested by determining the patient's ability to retain a slip of paper between the extended digits while the examiner attempts to withdraw the paper. Extension of the metacarpophalangeal joints against resistance applied to the proximal phalanges tests the extensors of the digits which are supplied by the radial nerve. The flexor digitorum sublimis muscle flexes the second phalanx of each finger and, by continued action, flexes the first phalanx. This muscle is supplied by the median nerve and may be tested in either of the following manners: (1) With all but the finger being tested held in full extension, only the flexor sublimis muscle to the finger being tested can flex the proximal interphalangeal joint. (2) With the wrist in a neutral position, the proximal phalanx of each finger is stabilized while the middle phalanx is flexed at the proximal interphalangeal joint against resistance applied to the middle phalanx. The distal phalanx should remain relaxed during this examination. This procedure is considered generally less satisfactory than the first one.

To test the flexor digitorum profundus muscle, which is supplied on the radial side by the median nerve and on the ulnar side by the ulnar nerve, the examiner holds the metacarpophalangeal and the proximal interphalangeal joints in rigid extension while the patient attempts to flex the distal phalanx of the finger. Because of the interconnections of the flexor tendons, the distal phalanx of one finger cannot be flexed strongly without the occurrence of flexion in the other distal interphalangeal joints. If slight motion is observed in the distal phalanges during this test, it results from the fixation or the tenodesis effect of tendons, fascia, and skin of the flexor aspect of the hand, or infrequently from an anomalous flexor digitorum profundus muscle which may have a separate muscle belly to the second (index) finger.

The strength of the three thumb muscles supplied by the median nerve can be tested by evaluating motion of the thumb with the following maneuvers: (1) Palmar abduction of the thumb (perpendicular to the plane of the palm) against resistance of the examiner's finger applied at the metacarpophalangeal joint tests the abductor pollicis brevis. (2) The flexor pollicis longus is tested by having the patient flex the distal interphalangeal joint against manual resistance applied by the examiner with the patient's thumb in palmar adduction while the metacarpophalangeal joint and proximal phalanx are stabilized by the examiner's other hand. (3) The opponens pollicis muscle can be tested by having the patient move his thumb across the palm and rotate the thumb into apposition with his fifth finger. While the patient keeps his thumb in apposition to, and in contact with, the fifth finger, the examiner attempts to rotate and draw the thumb back into its original position.

Suggested Reading for Additional Information

Refer to references at the end of Chapter 7, page 69.

CHAPTER NINE

THE SPINAL COLUMN

ESSENTIAL ANATOMY

Vertebrae
Atlas
Axis
Lumbosacral Portion
Sacro-iliac Articulation
Ligaments
Muscles
Surface Anatomy

INSPECTION

Spinal Curvatures

PALPATION AND PERCUSSION

Palpation
    Back
    Gluteal muscle attachments
    Fat pads and adipose tissue
Percussion

MOVEMENT AND RANGE OF MOTION

Methods of Determining Range of Motion
    Flexion
    Extension
    Lateral motion
    Rotation
    Cervical motion
    Costovertebral motion

SPECIAL EXAMINATIONS OF THE BACK

Supine Position
    Straight leg-raising test
    Rocking the pelvis
    Passive extension test
    Hyperextension of an extremity on the vertebral
        column
Prone Position
    Hyperextension of back
    Passive flexion of knee
Side Position
    Compression of iliac crests
Sitting Position
    Lumbar spinal motion
    Tests referable to the cervical vertebrae
    Warning concerning tests referable to cervical
        vertebrae

ADDITIONAL SPECIAL EXAMINATIONS

Digital Rectal Examination
    Palpation of piriformis muscle
    Palpation of the coccyx and sacrococcyx
Bimanual Pelvic Examination
Neurologic Examination

ESSENTIAL ANATOMY

The unique structure of the vertebral column allows flexibility of the trunk and also helps retain an upright posture by means of the coordinated action of muscles, ligaments, and bones. The vertebral column normally has four curves, two with anterior convexities (one in the cervical and one in the lumbar region) and two with posterior convexities (one in the thorax and one in the sacrococcygeal region). The curved shape of the vertebral column and the normally resilient structure of the intervertebral disks help to absorb a substantial degree of shock or concussion. If the curves of the spine are balanced or compensatory as they are in the normal back, the upright position can be maintained with much less muscular effort than when these curves are not balanced or compensated.

Vertebrae

The structure of the vertebrae determines to a great extent the mechanics of the spinal column. A typical vertebra consists of an anterior portion known as the vertebral body and a posterior portion which is the vertebral arch. The vertebral body and adjacent disks are the weight-bearing portions. The size of the vertebral body varies with the weight it supports; it increases in size from the second cervical vertebra to the first portion of the sacrum and then diminishes in size to the tip of the coccyx as the total body weight is transmitted from the lower part of the spinal column to the bony pelvis and lower extremities.

The arches of the vertebrae enclose the spinal cord. Each side of a vertebral arch is formed by a pedicle and a lamina which extends from the pedicle. The laminae from the two sides fuse in the midline posteriorly to complete the posterior boundary of the arch. One bony posterior spinous process and a lateral process on each side, known as the transverse process, project from the laminae and are the sites of muscle attachments. The spinous process projects dorsally in the midline where its tip lies subcutaneously and is easily palpable except high in the cervical area. A caudad slant of the spinous process in the thoracic region places the tip of the process at a level opposite the body of the adjacent lower vertebra, but in the lumbar region the

99

spinous process is at a level with the lower portion of its corresponding body. The transverse processes project on each side from the region of the junction of the pedicle and lamina; these are not palpable.

The vertebral arch also supports articular processes which originate from the junctions of the pedicles and laminae. There are four for each vertebra, one projecting downward from each side of the vertebra and one projecting upward on each side of the vertebra to form true or diarthrodial joints between adjacent vertebrae. These joints, known as apophyseal joints and also referred to as articular facets, thus have articular cartilages, thin articular capsules, and synovial membranes. The contact established between the superior articular process of one vertebra with the inferior articular process of the next lower one stabilizes the movement of the vertebrae and particularly prevents forward displacement of a vertebra on the next lower one. The angle of the articular surfaces of the apophyseal joints in relation to the horizontal plane of the vertebral bodies varies at different levels and determines to a large degree the type, as well as the extent of, the movement allowed in various sections of the vertebral column.

The vertebral bodies also articulate with each other by means of a fibrocartilaginous intervertebral disk and thin cartilaginous plates which cover the superior and inferior surfaces of the vertebral body. The cartilaginous plate lies between the disk and the vertebral body. The outer or superficial layers of the intervertebral disk are composed of tough fibers arranged concentrically that form the nucleus fibrosus. The center of the disk (the nucleus pulposus) normally is filled with a soft, mucoid substance. The elasticity of the disks permits compression of one edge of the disk and compensatory expansion on the other side of the disk as well as some upward, downward, and rotatory motion between adjacent vertebral bodies. Movement between two adjacent vertebrae is greatest where the disk is thickest as in the cervical and lumbar regions, and least where the disk is thinnest as in the thoracic region. The elasticity of the disk provides a cushion or "shock-absorber" effect between adjacent vertebrae, distributes the weight of the body, and thereby prevents concentration of weight on any one edge when the vertebral column is not in an upright position. The disks are thicker ventrally than dorsally in the cervical and lumbar region, and thus contribute to formation of the normal curvature of the spinal column in these areas. Intervertebral disks constitute about one fourth of the total length of the vertebral column above the sacrum.

Atlas

The atlas or first cervical vertebra differs in structure from the other vertebrae in that it lacks a vertebral body and consists only of an anterior and a posterior arch and thickened lateral masses. The atlas is a ring of bone which encloses a central vertebral foramen. The anterior arch forms about one fifth of the circumference of the ring, and the posterior arch forms about two fifths of the circumference; the lateral masses make up the remaining two fifths. The transverse atlantal ligament stretches across the ring of the atlas and divides the vertebral foramen into two unequal parts. The anterior or smaller portion serves as a receptacle for the odontoid process of the axis; the posterior or larger portion encloses the spinal cord. The lateral masses of the atlas rest on the second cervical vertebra and also support the skull. The skull articulates with the atlas by two joints (the atlanto-occipital joints) formed by the occipital condyles, which project inferiorly on each side from the base of the skull, and the superior articular facets of the atlas, which are directed upward and medially from each lateral mass, forming a cup for the corresponding occipital condyle. These atlanto-occipital joints permit flexion and extension (nodding movements of the head) and slight lateral bending of the head on the neck but very little, if any, rotation of the skull on the atlas, the latter motion being a function of the axis.

Axis

The axis or second cervical vertebra differs from other vertebrae by having a projection from the upper portion of its vertebral body which is the dens or odontoid process. The axis articulates with the atlas through paired lateral joints and a midline joint formed between the odontoid process and the ring formed by the anterior arch and transverse ligament of the atlas. The midline joint (medial atlanto-axial joint) is a trichoid or pivot joint with two synovial cavities, one between the anterior arch of the atlas and the odontoid process and the other between the posterior surface of the odontoid and the transverse atlantal ligament. Each lateral joint also has an articular capsule and synovial membrane. These articulations permit rotation of the skull and atlas on the odontoid process.

Lumbosacral Portion

The lumbosacral junction is a point of transition between the movable and immovable portions of the spinal column and its anterior surface is more caudad than its posterior surface. This creates a sharp anteroposterior angulation at the lumbosacral junction that results in the exertion of considerable leverage in this region by the entire length of the vertebral column above the sacrum. A tendency for the fifth lumbar vertebra to sublux anteriorly on the first sacral vertebra as a result of this leverage is countered by the posterior apposition of the articular processes between the fifth lumbar vertebra and the first sacral

101

vertebra. The intervertebral disk at the lumbosacral joint usually is much thicker, especially anteriorly, than other disks and thus provides for extra compressibility as well as greater motion. Besides being particularly vulnerable to the effects of mechanical stresses, the lumbosacral portion of the vertebral column is also a relatively common site of congenital anomalies of the vertebrae and abnormalities of the intervertebral disks.

Sacro-iliac Articulation

The sacrum articulates with the bony pelvis of the skeleton by means of a sacro-iliac joint on each side of the sacrum. Through these joints the weight of the body above the sacrum is transmitted to the bony pelvis and lower extremities. The upper portion of the sacrum is wider than the lower portion. The sacrum appears to be wedged between the ilia, and its upper end extends farther forward than its lower end.

Each sacro-iliac joint is formed by the internal or medial surface of the ilium and the lateral aspect of the first, second, and third sacral vertebrae. The sacro-iliac joints have an articular capsule and a synovial membrane. The joint cavity is a narrow, irregular slit, and the articular surfaces of the sacrum and ilium are covered with a layer of cartilage. A series of strong but short intra-articular fibers (the interosseous sacro-iliac ligament) connect the tuberosities of the sacrum and ilium, filling the narrow space between these bones in the posterior portion of the joint. The sacro-iliac joints are stabilized by unusually strong, dense, extracapsular ligaments which resist the tendency of the upper end of the sacrum to rotate forward and the lower end of the sacrum to rotate backward during weight bearing on these joints. Generally, very little motion is present in these joints; what motion there is disappears with increasing age and usually is gone by middle age.

Ligaments

The vertebrae are bound together by the anterior and posterior longitudinal ligaments which extend from the sacrum to the base of the occiput. These ligaments greatly increase the stability of the vertebral column. The dense anterior longitudinal ligament is stronger than the posterior longitudinal ligament and limits extension of the vertebral column. The space between the laminae of two adjacent vertebrae is filled by the ligamenta flava, which are thick, paired plates of elastic tissue that help restore the vertebral column to its original position after bending movements. The spinous processes are connected by the supraspinous and interspinous ligaments which partially limit flexion and lateral bending of the vertebral column.

Muscles

The large superficial muscles of the back (the trapezius and the latissimus dorsi on each side) almost completely cover the deeper, intrinsic muscles of the back. The latter are composed of a superficial layer consisting of the splenius capitis, splenius cervicis and sacrospinalis muscles on each side and a deeper layer of smaller muscles including the semispinalis, multifidus, rotatores, interspinales, and intertransversarii on each side.

A layer or a sheet of lumbodorsal fascia covers the intrinsic muscles of the back and extends upward to the region of the neck where it becomes continuous with the nuchal fascia. The intrinsic muscles of the back normally function as a unit to control or counteract flexion by extending the vertebral column. The sacrospinalis, also known as the erector spinae, occupies a groove on each side of the spinous processes and extends from the sacrum to the upper cervical vertebrae and base of the skull. These muscles are the longest muscles in the back and are especially well developed and prominent in the lumbar region. Bilateral action of the sacrospinalis muscles counteracts flexion and produces extension or hyperextension of the vertebral column. Muscles attached to the anterior surface of the vertebrae such as the quadratus lumborum, psoas major, and psoas minor assist in flexion of the vertebral column. The muscles of the abdominal wall (external oblique, internal oblique, and rectus abdominis) also are important flexors of the spinal column. Abduction (lateral bending) and rotation of the spinal column are performed by contraction of these abdominal and intrinsic back muscles on one side with simultaneous relaxation of the comparable muscles on the opposite side.

Surface Anatomy

Certain easily identified and normally present surface landmarks are useful for orientation in the examination of the back. The spinous processes of the seventh cervical and first thoracic vertebrae are especially prominent in the midline at the base of the back of the neck. The inferior angle of the scapula normally lies at the level of, and lateral to, the interspace between the seventh and eighth thoracic vertebrae. The iliac crest is easily palpable from the posterior to the anterior iliac spines. A line joining the highest point on each iliac crest crosses the body of the fourth lumbar vertebra. The prominences of the spinous processes are usually readily palpable at the bottom of a furrow which runs down the midline of the back from the external occipital protuberance to the middle of the sacrum. On each side of this furrow is a rounded elevation produced by the sacrospinalis muscle. In the sacral region the furrow becomes shallower, forming a flattened triangular area whose apex lies on the gluteal cleft. The sides of this triangle originate from two symmetrical dimples that overlie the posterior superior iliac spines. A line connecting the posterior superior iliac spines crosses the body of the second sacral vertebra. The midportion of each sacro-iliac joint lies adjacent and medial to the posterior superior iliac spine on the same side. The upper border of the gluteus maximus muscle arises about 3 cm. lateral to the posterior superior iliac spine and runs along the iliac crest; its fibers extend downward and laterally to the prominence of the greater trochanter. A line drawn horizontally at the level of the ischial tuberosities crosses the femurs at the level of the lesser trochanters. The tip of the coccyx lies above the level of the ischial tuberosities.

INSPECTION

Inspection of the back should be made after the patient has removed all clothing, including shoes. The entire back, thighs, legs, hips, and shoulders should be visible. The patient may be draped with a sheet or gown which does not prevent this. When possible, the patient should stand erect with feet together, hips and knees extended, and arms hanging at the sides. The examiner should be far enough away from the patient to permit an initial inspection of the whole back.

Spinal Curvatures

The patient is inspected from behind, from the side, and from the front. From behind, it should be noted whether or not the spine is abnormally curved to one or the other side (scoliosis) or whether there is an exaggeration or flattening of normal anteroposterior curves. A list or tilting of the trunk of the body to one side is present when an imaginary vertical line indicates that the prominence of the spinous process of the first thoracic vertebra is not centered over the midline of the sacrum. The degree of list is measured by the deviation of such an imaginary perpendicular line from the prominence of the posterior spinous process of the first thoracic vertebra to a region lateral to the gluteal cleft, but it may be obscured by compensatory curves. Compensation for scoliosis or lateral curvature of the spinal column is complete when the first thoracic vertebra is centered over the sacrum, regardless of the curvature between these points. Scoliosis is described according to the direction of its convexity. Thus, left lumbar scoliosis would have a convexity of the lumbar curve to the left. Scoliosis may be further defined as functional or structural in type. Functional scoliosis such as that due to a significant shortening of one leg will be present when the patient is in the upright position but will disappear when the patient bends forward. This is in contrast to structural scoliosis which does not disappear in the flexed position and may even be accentuated in this position in comparison to the upright position. Scoliosis in the thoracic region may produce a rotation of the vertebrae which results in a hump or prominence ("gibbus") of the thorax on the side of the convexity. Scoliosis in the lumbar region usually is associated with a prominence of the sacrospinalis muscle on the side of the convexity, but deformity due to a prominence of the vertebrae is less evident in the lumbar region than in the thoracic region. Palpation of the spinous processes is often necessary to confirm the presence or absence of an abnormal spinal curvature suspected from inspection of the back.

A lateral tilt of the pelvis may be observed by comparing the level of the iliac crests when the patient is standing. Normally the superior iliac crests are level, but when the pelvis is tilted laterally, one iliac crest is higher than the other. If the pelvis is tilted to one side, scoliosis is usually present with the convexity facing toward the low side. When a lateral curvature of the spinal column is present and the iliac crests remain level, the deviation of the vertebral column originates within the column itself and cannot be attributed to causes producing a pelvic tilt. When a pelvic tilt and associated scoliosis are caused by a short leg, both can be eliminated by having the patient stand during the examination with a block of wood or other supports (such as magazines or books of various thicknesses) under the short leg.

Paravertebral muscles in spasm tend to stand out as delineated muscle masses which are visible on inspection; the muscles look as though they were being pushed out from beneath the skin on one or both sides of the spinous processes. Paravertebral muscle spasm may be more prominent on one side than the other and is often associated with spasm of the muscles forming the buttock on the involved side (Fig. 73). This is relatively common in patients with sciatic pain secondary to a protruded lumbar disk. Asymmetry of the skin folds in the gluteal region may reveal a pelvic tilt or shortness of a lower extremity as described on page 130 in the chapter on "The Hip."

The presence of subcutaneous fibrous-tissue nodules also should be noted. Such nodules are found most often over bony prominences (Fig. 74).

When the patient is standing and is being inspected from the side, the vertebral column has a characteristic thoracic kyphosis (posterior curvature) and a lumbar lordosis (anterior curvature). An increase or decrease from normal of these curves should be observed. The vertebral column tends to balance anterior and posterior curves; thus, an increase in lumbar lordosis is frequently accompanied by an increase in thoracic kyphosis or vice versa. Posture may be altered by an increase

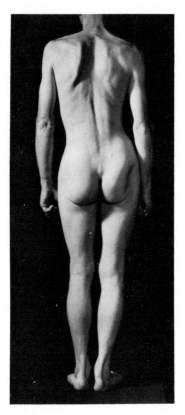

Figure 73. Posterior view of the back showing marked paravertebral muscle spasm which is particularly prominent on the right side and is associated with spasm of the muscles forming the right buttock. A thoracolumbar scoliosis is present with the convexity on the left. The right shoulder is lower than the left. A pelvic tilt is present with the right hip held high. The gluteal skin folds are slightly elevated on the right side. The patient had bilateral sciatica, but it was more marked on the right side and resulted from a midline and right-sided protrusion of the fourth lumbar intervertebral disk.

or decrease of chest development, rounding of the shoulders, protuberance of the abdomen, forward protuberance of the head, and varying degrees of forward tilting of the pelvis (Fig. 75). These variations also are noted during inspection from the side.

Observation of the patient from the front for evidence of abnormalities associated with involvement of the spinal column completes inspection of the spine. If the patient is draped with a sheet or gown, the drape should be removed or drawn to the midline to permit adequate inspection of spinal abnormalities. Nutritional status, general body type, symmetry or asymmetry of trunk or extremities, position of the head and neck, and the level of the nipples and shoulders are sometimes more evident in this view, but actual structural abnormalities of the spinal column are best determined from the lateral or posterior views. The patient's gait should be observed from the front, the side, and the back.

PALPATION AND PERCUSSION

Palpation and percussion of the back may produce pain or reveal tenderness of abnormal structures. However, since abnormalities of differ-

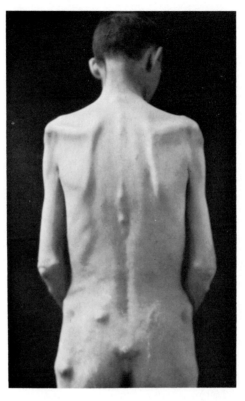

Figure 74. Multiple sub-cutaneous rheumatoid nodules over bony prominences on back, pelvis, and hips.

ent structures in the back may produce similar symptoms, it is important that the examiner evaluate these structures in a systematic fashion and recheck positive findings to confirm initial impressions. Pain or tenderness during palpation or percussion of the back may originate as follows: 1. Abnormalities of joints and adjacent bones may produce pain or localized tenderness. For example, low back pain may result from involvement of the sacro-iliac joints, degenerative changes in the lumbar vertebrae, or a localized destructive process in a vertebra or intervertebral disk. 2. Muscle spasm in the region of the back is a common source of pain and may make evaluation of underlying structures by palpation or percussion difficult or even impossible. Muscle spasm may result from degenerative or inflammatory processes in muscle fibers or, secondarily, from misuse of muscles resulting in sustained contractions. It also is seen often in chronic or acute anxiety states. Secondary muscle spasm may accompany painful lesions in structures adjacent to involved muscles and sometimes produces tenderness along the sites of muscle attachments to bones. 3. Referred nerve pain, which often is transient and shooting but may be persistent, characteristically occurs along the distribution of a particular nerve root. An example is sciatic nerve pain which accompanies a protruded intervertebral disk in the

107

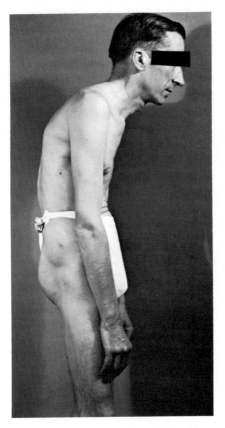

Figure 75. Lateral view of patient with ankylosing (rheumatoid) spondylitis showing forward protrusion of head, flattening of anterior chest wall, thoracic kyphosis, protrusion of abdomen, and flattening of lumbar lordosis. This patient also has slight flexion of the hips on the pelvis. (Reprinted from Hench, P. S., Slocumb, C. H., and Polley, H. F.: Rheumatoid Spondylitis: Questions and Answers. M. Clin. North America, July, 1947, p. 885, Fig. 149.)

lumbar region. This type of pain occurs even when adjacent muscles are relaxed. Referred pain to the back from abdominal visceral diseases usually produces pain and muscle spasm localized to one spot in the distribution of the affected nerve arc. 4. Low back pain also may result from tenderness of localized soft-tissue structures such as fat pads, ligaments, and tissues overlying bony structures such as spinous processes.

Palpation

Back. Palpation of the back while the patient is standing, lying prone, and sitting provides information that supplements the findings on palpation in any one position. When a patient is tense or muscle spasm is present, palpation is more satisfactory when the patient is prone than in any other position. A pillow under the abdomen to support the spinal column is desirable; the pillow not only flattens the lumbar lordosis but also separates the spinous processes so that they can be identified more easily.

Palpation of the back is performed with the examiner's fingertips and thumbs. The patient is directed to point out areas of tenderness or discomfort as specifically as possible before the examination is started. The diffuseness or specificity of such subjective localization can be of considerable significance when correlated with the physical findings. During palpation, the findings are noted in reference to the anatomic landmarks of the back just described. Palpation of subcutaneous tissues in an area removed from the patient's localization of discomfort helps to accustom the patient to the examination and enables the examiner to evaluate the patient's pain threshold and general demeanor and reactivity as well as the tone of muscles and the subcutaneous turgor. Areas of localized tenderness not previously described by the patient may be found and the presence of any local heat, nodules, fat pads, or masses should be noted.

In general, palpation is performed from the top downward or vice versa and from side to side at various levels. The posterior aspect of the vertebral column is palpated for evidence of abnormal prominence of any spinous process; this may indicate a collapsed vertebral body from mechanical, metabolic, infectious, inflammatory, or malignant disease. A bony shelf or abnormal projection of one vertebra in relation to its adjacent vertebrae suggests subluxation or spondylolisthesis. Any other bony irregularities should be palpated; these are especially prominent at the lumbosacral level and in the regions of the spinous processes, scapulae, and shoulder girdle. When palpation over the attachments of the gluteal muscle and the lumbosacral joints reveals muscles in spasm, the muscles are likely to be tender and feel abnormally tight and contracted.

Excessive muscle spasm produces pain and tenderness in the distribution of the involved muscle. In such instances the original site of pain often cannot be determined accurately until the muscle has been relaxed. It may be necessary in such instances to re-examine the patient after a period of rest in bed when a more comfortable position can be attained. When excessive spasm exists, it is best to defer conclusive evaluation of the spinal examination until it can be performed more reliably.

Gluteal Muscle Attachments. Tenderness of the gluteal muscle attachments also can be evaluated best with the patient lying on his abdomen. Palpation is carried out with the leg in active hyperextension. The patient is directed to raise his leg (with the knee extended) high enough off the table to cause contraction and tightening of the gluteal muscles in order to exert a pull on muscle attachments, but the leg should not be raised high enough to mobilize the pelvis or lumbar vertebrae since disorders of these structures may produce symptoms and thus prevent localization of pain. If the gluteal muscle attachments are involved, this maneuver should reproduce the patient's pain and localized palpation over the superior attachments of the gluteal muscles will help differentiate this pain from other sites of subcutaneous tenderness.

Fat Pads and Adipose Tissue. These may be the sites of localized tenderness, especially in the gluteal muscle and lumbosacral regions. The tenderness may be localized or may involve adipose tissues more diffusely. Fat pads or adipose tissue can be evaluated best by picking up these tissues between the examiner's finger and thumb and palpating them specifically for tenderness. Tender areas can be evaluated further by the examiner's moving the skin and superficial fatty tissues to one side with one hand, while palpating underlying structures with the other hand. If the underlying structures are not tender, the tenderness that has been demonstrated previously must involve the superficial tissues that have been moved aside by the examiner.

Percussion

Percussion is performed over the vertebrae and spinous processes in both painless and painful areas to appraise the patient's tolerance of discomfort. Examination by percussion should include the lumbosacral joint, sacro-iliac joints, spinous processes, and the sacral attachments of the latissimus dorsi. As with palpation, this can be done from the top downward or vice versa and from side to side, but in any event percussion should be performed systematically to avoid omission of any particular area.

Mild jarring of the spinous processes with the ulnar aspect of the examiner's fist may reveal generalized or localized tenderness but does not distinguish between the pain of muscle spasm and the pain of intrinsic disease or abnormality of bony structures. When generalized tenderness is found by this means, more accurate localization should be attempted by careful percussion of the region with the tip of the examiner's third (middle) finger. If the examiner's third (middle) finger is placed over a spinous process and percussed while the second and fourth fingers of the same hand are placed on either side of the spine, paravertebral muscle spasm may be readily detected and localized for the reaction detected by the second and fourth fingers. Pain which is accompanied by muscle spasm prevents accurate localization, but localized pain in the absence of muscle spasm often represents a significant abnormality of the structures in the area being examined. The use of the three fingers spaced apart as described also permits more accurate localization of painful areas detected by percussion.

Jarring of the spinal column can be accomplished also by having the patient rise from the standing position to stand on his toes and then forcibly drop back to the floor on his heels. This type of percussion maneuver may indicate in general whether the pain or tenderness is present in the spinal region and occasionally helps in the localization of pain; however, usually more specific localized percussion as described is required.

MOVEMENT AND RANGE OF MOTION

The vertebral column permits extension (bending backward), flexion (bending forward), abduction (bending to either side), and rotation. The extent of these movements varies in different regions of the vertebral column. Movement of the spinal column is greatest in the cervical region, is more restricted in the lumbar and thoracic regions, and is not present in the sacral region. Mobility in the vertebral column depends primarily on the thickness and elasticity of the intervertebral disks, the position and direction of the interarticular facets, and the limitations established by the vertebral ligaments. Age, general physical condition, and previous or unusual physical activity are also significant factors that affect spinal movement. Spinal mobility varies considerably among normal individuals. Movement of the vertebral column as a whole should be differentiated from movement which takes place primarily in certain segments such as the cervical or lumbar regions. Forward bending usually includes both flexion of the hips and of the vertebral column, and it is difficult to separate the two components without fixation of the pelvis by the examiner in order to assess just the range of spinal flexion. The values used to assess the range of spinal motion generally are only approximations for adults up to middle age. There is a tendency for spinal mobility to decrease somewhat after middle age.

Flexion occurs primarily in the cervical, low thoracic, and lumbar regions. Flexion of the vertebral column as a whole produces the greatest range of motion. From the neutral or upright position, the column as a whole usually flexes to about 90 degrees. If the cervical portion is not included in the movement and the pelvis is stabilized, the trunk flexes about 40 degrees.

Extension of the vertebral column takes place mainly in the cervical and lumbar regions. If the cervical portion is not included in the measurement, the trunk extends about 30 degrees from the neutral or upright position.

In order to maintain balance, the pelvis normally shifts in the opposite direction as the trunk moves backward or forward.

The vertebral column as a whole bends about 60 degrees to either side; this occurs mostly in the cervical, low thoracic, and lumbar regions. If cervical motion is excluded, lateral motion of the low thoracic and lumbar portions is about 20 degrees to each side.

Rotation is most marked in the cervical region and is relatively restricted in the lumbar and thoracic regions. If motion of the neck is excluded and the pelvis is stabilized, the vertebral column rotates about 30 degrees to each side.

111

Methods of Determining Range of Motion

Spinal motion is determined from the positions used for inspection. When the examiner is seated behind the standing patient, he can stabilize the patient's extremities by adducting his own knees and legs against the patient's legs and thus can detect or prevent any movement of the patient's legs during examination of motion of the vertebral column. Spinal bending should be performed without permitting the patient to bend his knees or hips. When the examiner is standing behind or alongside the patient, he can stabilize the patient's hips and pelvis by holding the pelvis firmly with his hands and arms in a hugging type of grasp while the patient bends forward.

Flexion. When bending forward, the patient should flex his head and neck as well as the other segments of the vertebral column and let his arms hang at the sides of his body or fall forward with the bending motion. With the motion of this maneuver the lumbar lordotic curve normally will first flatten and then flex slightly, as the amount of forward bending increases. Normally, the flexed position when viewed from the side forms a smooth curve extending from the sacrum to the base of the skull (Fig. 76). A persistent flattening or lordosis of the lumbar

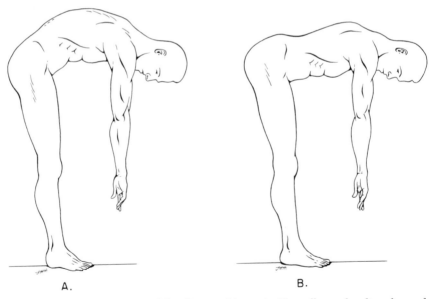

A.   B.

Figure 76. Forward bending positions. A. Normally on bending forward the entire spinal column has a smooth curved contour when viewed from the side. B. A persistence of the lumbar lordotic curve while bending forward indicates limitation of functional motion in the lumbar vertebrae. Note that the motion of flexion is all taking place in the hip joints. This abnormality is characteristic of conditions associated with marked spasm of paravertebral muscles.

region while the patient is bending forward indicates an abnormal loss of motion in this portion of the spinal column. Whether this abnormality is intrinsic or from muscle spasm can often be best evaluated by viewing the spinal column from the side. Abnormal prominences or sharp angulations of the vertebral column also may be detected from a side view.

Normal spinal flexion is a straightforward motion. Lateral or rotatory deviations during flexion usually indicate asymmetric muscle spasm but do not indicate the reason for the spasm.

Movement of the spinal column also may be evaluated by palpation of the separation of the lumbar spinous processes, which normally occurs during flexion. This is accomplished when the examiner places two or more fingers of one hand on adjacent spinous processes and observes the range of spread of the fingers during spinal flexion. Failure of the spinous processes to separate indicates limitation of motion.

The degree of spinal flexion plus flexion of the hips is often recorded by measuring the distance from the fingertips to the floor, specifying the number of inches ahead of the toes that is used for the site of the measurement. However, if only the range of spinal motion is being determined, this is not accurate. Various graphic devices or arbitrary grading systems also can be used to record range of spinal motion, but careful measurement of height without shoes is a satisfactorily accurate method of determining changes in spinal curves or motions in an individual patient over a period of time.

Extension.   The degree of extension of the vertebral column is determined by having the patient bend backward. During this motion, the patient stands with both feet on the floor and the examining physician stabilizes the pelvis by firm pressure with his fist against the patient's sacrum and by counter pressure with his other hand on the upper anterior portion of one of the patient's thighs. Normally the trunk will extend about 30 degrees from the upright position. Extension usually increases the lordotic lumbar curve, straightens out the thoracic part of the vertebral column, and tilts the head backward. Failure to increase the lordotic lumbar curve indicates limitation of motion in this portion of the spinal column. The degree of spinal extension can be measured by various graphic devices, or spinal motion can be estimated by percentages of normalcy or arbitrary grades.

Lateral Motion.   Lateral motion of the spinal column is determined when the patient bends to one side and then the other. Lateral motion can be observed in a manner similar to that described for spinal flexion, but if the patient stands with his feet about 20 to 24 inches apart and keeps the knees fully extended, the pelvis is more satisfactorily stabilized for lateral bending than if the feet are close together. The normal spinal column has a smooth, lateral curve of about 60 degrees from the upright position extending from the sacrum to the base of the skull. Sharp angulations, pain, and muscle spasm during

113

lateral spinal motion as well as during flexion and extension are abnormal and should be noted. Normally the degree of lateral motion is equal on both sides; inequality of motion indicates functional restriction of motion on one side. When the arc of the curve of the spinal column is greater while the patient is bending to one side than it is while he is bending to the other, abnormal movement is also indicated.

Rotation. This is evaluated when the patient rotates the trunk to one side and then the other while his legs and pelvis are stabilized. Rotation takes place primarily in the thoracic and cervical regions. The trunk can rotate about 90 degrees to either side; however, if neck motion is excluded and the pelvis is stabilized, the low thoracic and lumbar portions rotate only about 30 degrees to either side.

Cervical Motion. This is evaluated in either the standing or the sitting position. The patient tips his head forward for flexion, backward for extension, and for rotation turns his head to each side as if looking over each shoulder. Lateral motion is determined when the patient tries to touch his ear to his shoulder without raising the shoulder girdle. Normally the cervical portion of the spine allows about 45 degrees of flexion, 50 to 60 degrees of extension, 60 to 80 degrees of rotation, and 40 degrees of lateral bending. The atlanto-occipital joint permits most of the motions of flexion and extension, and the atlanto-axial joint permits rotation. Lateral motion of the neck occurs primarily below the atlas from the motions of the second to seventh cervical vertebrae. Thus, the specific limitation of the neck observed indicates the part of the cervical spinal column involved.

The location of neck pain which occurs during lateral cervical motion may be of considerable help in differentiating pain from muscle spasm from that due to involvement of the spinal apophyseal joints. When pain is reproduced on the same side toward which the neck is tilted, involvement of the apophyseal joints is suggested since this motion compresses the articular facets on the same side, thereby aggravating any already existing irritation of the nerve roots. By contrast, when neck pain occurs on the side opposite the one toward which the neck is rotated, muscle pain is suggested since the muscles on the opposite side of the neck are stretched by this motion.

Costovertebral Motion. This is determined by measuring chest expansion during inspiration and expiration. This may be estimated by inspection of the act of deep inspiration and expiration from the back and sides while the examiner's hands are placed on either side of the lower posterolateral portion of the thorax; expansion of the chest thus can be both seen and felt. However, measurement of chest expansion with a nonelastic tape measure is easy and is the only accurate method of measurement. Different absolute measurements of the chest expansion will be found at various levels of the thorax and may account for differences noted by different examiners if this factor is not considered.

114

The nipple line (or just above it in females) is a generally satisfactory and recommended standard site for measurement of chest expansion. The degree of chest expansion, like other spinal motions, varies with age and general physical condition, but normally it is at least 5 to 6 cm. in young adults but may be up to 10 to 13 cm. in some individuals.

SPECIAL EXAMINATIONS OF THE BACK

Many types of special examinations of the vertebral column have been described. Although one or more of these special tests may aid in establishing the correct diagnosis, single special tests are usually not specific enough to be diagnostic or completely reliable in establishing either the site or nature of the lesion. Likewise a single test, especially if it is negative, often does not exclude the particular condition for which the test has been proposed.

Certain special tests discussed next are grouped according to the position of the patient in which they are performed.

Supine Position

Straight Leg-Raising Test. This test is carried out by the examiner while the patient's leg and thigh are as relaxed as is possible. The examiner places one hand under the patient's heel and holds the foot firmly in dorsiflexion by exerting pressure cephalad from this grasp. While the examiner gradually and passively flexes the thigh on the pelvis by motion of the foot, the examiner's other hand is placed just above the patella of the side being tested and with it he exerts gentle but firm downward pressure to hold the knee fully extended. The limit of the angle of flexion is measured by the degrees in the angle formed between the surface on which the patient is lying and the elevated lower extremity. The patient's other leg and thigh should be stabilized in extension while this test is being performed. The angle at which pain, muscle spasm, or flexion of the pelvis occurs is compared with that observed on similar examination of the opposite lower extremity.

Elevation of the lower extremity produces tension on the sciatic nerve and hamstring muscles, but normally each leg and thigh can be raised to almost a right angle without discomfort. When this examination causes pain in the region of the hip or low in the back and limitation of flexion at the hip in the extremity being examined, the test is considered "positive" and suggests nerve root irritation or muscle spasm on the painful side. Straight leg raising flattens the lumbar part of the vertebral column, stretches the ligaments and extensor muscles of the hip and thigh and thus may suggest an abnormality of the lumbosacral or sacro-iliac regions rather than of the sciatic nerve. Occasionally,

115

the straight leg raising test will produce pain in the sacral, gluteal, or posterior thigh regions on the side opposite to the one being examined. This also suggests nerve root irritation on the painful side. When this occurs, straight raising of the other leg also will cause pain in the same area. Mild discomfort behind the knee may be described by the patient due to tightening of the hamstrings or disease of the knee or popliteal area, but this should not be considered a positive response to the test.

When restriction of motion is observed, it is helpful for the examiner to perform the straight leg-raising test slowly with one hand and to palpate muscle spasm and movement of the spinal column with his other hand that is placed under the patient's lower vertebrae. If pain and muscle spasm occur low in the back before spinal movement is detected, a sacro-iliac lesion is suggested. Pain after motion of the lumbar vertebrae is compatible with either lumbosacral or sacro-iliac involvement.

Rocking the Pelvis. A form of passive movement of the lower part of the spinal column can be tested as follows: The examiner or the patient partially flexes the patient's knees; then the examiner grasps both the patient's legs with one arm under both thighs. The patient's thighs and lower part of the spinal column are flexed maximally, bringing both knees as close to the abdomen as possible. With the patient's legs in this position, the patient's pelvis is moved from side to side and also rotated back and forth on the spinal column by the examiner. Normally this rocking motion of the pelvis is painless. Thus the presence and location of pain resulting from either lateral or rotatory motions may be helpful in detecting and localizing significant involvement of the lumbar and lumbosacral portions of the spinal column. This maneuver also may produce or accentuate sciatic pain and hence should always be performed with caution.

Passive Extension Test. To perform this test, the patient is moved to one end of the examining table so that the patient's pelvis is at the edge of the table and the legs can be dropped down over the end of the table. When the leg on the involved side is lowered, pain develops in the sacral, gluteal, or posterior thigh region and is relieved by flexion of the unaffected leg while the affected leg is still down. Many lesions of the back or fascial contractures of the anterior portion of the thigh may cause some localized pain with this maneuver, but the procedure is of most significance when sciatic pain is present and sciatic radiation results from the maneuver.

Hyperextension of an Extremity on the Vertebral Column. To test more specifically for abnormality of the *sacro-iliac joints*, the patient is moved to one side of the examining table so that he lies with one leg and buttock close enough to this edge that the extremity can be let down over the side of the table to produce hyperextension of this extremity on the vertebral column. During this test the patient's pelvis and lumbar spine are held in a fixed position by having the patient grasp the extremity not being dropped over the side of the table just below the knee and with clasped hands having him flex the hip so that the thigh lies as much as possible against the abdomen. The examiner assists in this fixation of the patient's pelvis and lumbar vertebrae by placing one hand over the patient's clasped hands after the hip joint has been flexed. With the other hand the examiner then lowers the patient's leg on the side being examined so that both the leg and the thigh project over the edge of the table and gradually hyperextend the hip joint as far as possible.

The procedure is repeated for the other extremity by having the patient move across the examining table so that the opposite extremity can be dropped over the side of the table after fixation of the spinal column and pelvis, as just described. If the sacro-iliac joint is the site of pain, this maneuver accentuates the pain in the region of the sacro-iliac joint on the side of the hyperextended thigh. The test may be positive for unilateral or bilateral involvement of the sacro-iliac joints.

Prone Position

Hyperextension of Back. This test should be performed with the patient's arms in adduction and at the sides of his body with the palms of the hands next to the thighs in the resting position. The patient is instructed to raise his head, shoulders, and arms from the examining table as in arching or hyperextending the spinal column. The examiner stabilizes the patient's legs by exerting downward pressure with his hands on the thighs during this maneuver. The patient then relaxes and, after assuming the resting position again, is instructed to keep one leg extended while actively hyperextending each leg in sequence. These procedures may help the patient and the examiner to localize painful areas in the back to either bone or muscle. When the localization is referable to muscles, the pain produced by active hyperextension of the back by this maneuver is primarily in the attachment of the latissimus dorsi muscle, whereas the pain resulting from active hyperextension of the leg as described is primarily in attachments of the gluteus maximus muscles. It is advisable not to perform hyperextension of the back vigorously unless x-ray examination of this region has been obtained since this maneuver may aggravate intrinsic bony lesions.

A procedure for evaluating tenderness of the gluteal muscle attachments also was described on page 109 in the section on palpation of the back. It should be mentioned that active hyperextension of the leg in the prone position is painful when the *psoas muscle* is abnormal on the side of the elevated leg.

Useful information concerning *painful muscle spasm* in the back can be obtained sometimes when the examiner raises both of the patient's legs off the table by placing one arm under the legs at the level of the knees (or just above the knees if necessary for adequate leverage) and palpates the lower portion of the back and spinal column with his other hand. If the patient pushes down on the examiner's arm that is being used to elevate the lower extremities by attempting to flex his thighs, more complete relaxation of paravertebral and gluteal muscles may be obtained. This maneuver shortens the intrinsic muscles of the back and helps relieve muscle tension and spasm; it permits more accurate localization of tenderness by palpation with the hand that is not being used to raise the lower extremities. This maneuver may relieve pain due to muscle spasm in this area. Its principal value is in the possible assistance that may result from relaxation of muscle spasm which in turn permits better localization of tender areas in the lumbar and lumbosacral regions, especially when soft-tissue structures are involved. However, since this maneuver may aggravate intrinsic, mechanical disease of the spinal column, it is not advisable to use it when an osseous spinal lesion is suspected. In doubtful instances, it is best to defer this maneuver until roentgenograms of this area have been obtained.

Passive Flexion of Knee. This may aggravate pain in the lower part of the back and help to localize the site of pain, but it is not a specific test for any particular spinal or paraspinal lesion. Each extremity is tested separately and the knee is flexed as far as possible. When the knee is flexed fully to bring the heel to the buttock, disease in the lumbosacral region may cause pain and muscle spasm near the site of involvement. This maneuver may cause the pelvis or lumbar vertebrae to be lifted a few inches off the table, if the thighs are partially flexed in an attempt to relieve the pain and muscle spasm.

Side Position

Compression of Iliac Crests. This is produced by firm, sustained downward pressure with the examiner's hands for about half a minute over the upper iliac crest on the side opposite from that on which the patient is lying. Pain produced in the region of the *sacro-iliac joint* is a positive response that may be demonstrated by performing this test while the patient is lying on either the involved or uninvolved side. A positive response suggests sacro-iliac localization of the condition, but a negative response (no localization of pain during pressure) does not exclude sacro-iliac disease.

Sitting Position

Lumbar Spinal Motion. Examination of lumbar spinal motion when the patient is in the sitting position may reduce or eliminate any influence of the hip joints or hamstring muscles, and the findings obtained from tests carried out with the patient in this position can be compared with those obtained while the patient was standing. When the sacro-iliac joints are abnormal, forward bending from the sitting position may be freer than that observed in the standing position because the gluteal and hamstring muscles which also may be involved by the sacro-iliac disease are more relaxed. When there is an abnormality at the lumbosacral junction, diffuse muscle spasm or spinal fusion, forward bending from the sitting position remains as limited as it was from the standing position. The interpretation of these findings is seldom precise, but sometimes these maneuvers may be of differential value.

Tests Referable to the Cervical Vertebrae. Raising the skull up from the neck by *manual traction* may be a helpful procedure for evaluation of symptoms in the region of the cervical vertebrae. The examiner stands in front of the sitting patient and places the thenar eminence of each hand on each cheek just below the patient's maxilla and the finger tips of each hand firmly against the occiput on each side. Upward and inward pressure is applied firmly, slowly, steadily, and equally with both hands. Maximal manual traction is achieved with about 20 to 50 pounds (9 to 23 kg.) pull but should always be painless. The examiner's pressure is then slowly relieved, and the patient's head is carefully permitted to resume the position present before the test was started. It is advisable to explain the test to the patient in advance in order to obtain better relaxation and cooperation. Relief of possible radicular symptoms during manual traction suggests nerve root irritation at or near the intervertebral foramina, although muscle spasm also may be relieved temporarily by this maneuver.

Application of manual pressure to the top of a patient's head may reproduce or aggravate cervical radicular pain. It is more likely to reproduce the patient's symptoms if the pressure is applied while the patient's head is tilted toward the side of the involvement or when the neck is hyperextended. These maneuvers may be of differential value; however, it is advisable not to attempt them until an x-ray examination of the cervical vertebrae has excluded metastatic or osteoporotic disease of the vertebrae, subluxations or fractures of the cervical vertebrae or of the odontoid process or other bone or cord lesions which would contraindicate these procedures.

Warning Concerning Tests Referable to Cervical Vertebrae. Subluxation of the atlanto-axial articulation may cause radicular pain extending into the occipital region or into the arms or may produce extrinsic pressure on the spinal cord with bizarre neurologic symptoms below this level. Pain may be aggravated by sudden head movements or when the vertebral column is jarred. The patient may also have some difficulty in restoring the head to its normal position after looking

119

downward. This condition will be apparent from roentgenographic views of the cervical vertebrae including flexion and extension views, but when these symptoms are present, manipulation of the neck must be avoided.

ADDITIONAL SPECIAL EXAMINATIONS

Digital Rectal Examination

This examination is an essential part of the examination of the back. It is performed best when the patient's hips are flexed, and this can be accomplished with the patient in either a kneeling or a Trendelenburg position. The midportion of the sacro-iliac joint lies just below and lateral to the promontory of the sacrum and often is palpable on the rectal examination. The lower aspect of the sacro-iliac joint forms part of the upper edge of the sacrosciatic notch. Bimanual palpation of this region may be performed with the examiner's index finger in the rectum and the other hand placed externally over the lower portion of the back. Tenderness if localized to the sacro-iliac joint may be more evident on internal palpation, but a marked discrepancy between tenderness palpated rectally and externally is unusual with sacro-iliac involvement and should be noted if present. The examiner's finger in the rectum may be able to palpate sponginess or localize the presence of swelling or tenderness in the sacro-iliac region on either side. Palpation of the sacro-iliac area on rectal examination is limited by the proximity of the ischial tuberosities and thus is accomplished more satisfactorily in women than in men.

Palpation of Piriformis Muscle. It is also possible to palpate the piriformis muscle during rectal examination. The piriformis is a flat, pyramidal-shaped muscle which arises from the front of the sacrum where it is attached to portions of the first, second, third, and fourth sacral vertebrae and passes out of the pelvis through the greater sciatic foramen on each side to become inserted into the upper border of each greater trochanter. Localized tenderness or spasm in this muscle may cause pain in the buttocks, and pressure over this muscle on rectal examination may produce definite pain and discomfort. A painful piriformis muscle also can be localized if the hip on the involved side is flexed and the knee is extended during the rectal examination.

Palpation of the Coccyx and Sacrococcyx. The coccyx and sacrococcyx are also examined by palpation rectally and bimanually as described above for the sacro-iliac joints. The coccyx may be manipulated by the finger in the rectum and the thumb outside to evaluate angulation and mobility, and to localize tenderness on palpation or motion or both.

120

Bimanual Pelvic Examination

This examination is indicated in female patients to evaluate the lower spinal segments and the possible relation of pelvic organs thereto. The reader is referred to gynecologic texts for more details with regard to the technic of this examination and the interpretation of backache due to abnormalities of the pelvic organs. Backache is not commonly caused by disease of pelvic organs.

Neurologic Examination

Such an examination may be a necessary and integral part of the evaluation of the spinal column. The details of this examination can be found in neurologic texts and also are beyond the scope of this publication.

Suggested Reading for Additional Information

1. Schmorl, Georg, and Junghanns, Herbert: The Human Spine in Health and Disease. New York, Grune & Stratton, Inc., 1959, 285 pp.
2. Willis, T. A.: Man's Back. Springfield, Illinois, Charles C Thomas, Publisher, 1953, 161 pp.
3. Lewin, Philip: Backache and Sciatic Neuritis: Back Injuries, Deformities, Disabilities. Philadelphia, Lea & Febiger, 1943, 745 pp.
4. Hollinshead, W. H.: Anatomy for Surgeons. New York, Paul B. Hoeber, Inc., 1958, vol. 3, pp. 82–206.
5. Wilson, P. D., Jr.: Low Back Pain and Sciatica. In Hollander, J. L.: Arthritis and Allied Conditions: A Textbook of Rheumatology. Ed. 6, Philadelphia, Lea & Febiger, 1960, pp. 1235–1285.
6. Jackson, Ruth: The Cervical Syndrome. Ed. 2, Springfield, Illinois, Charles C Thomas, Publisher, 1958, 197 pp.
7. Polley, H. F.: The Diagnosis and Treatment of Rheumatoid Spondylitis. M. Clin. North America, 1955, pp. 509–528.
8. American Academy of Orthopaedic Surgeons: Measuring and Recording of Joint Motion. Everett, Massachusetts, Glenwood Press, 1963, 91 pp.
9. Novak, E. R., and Jones, Georgeanna S.: Textbook of Gynecology. Ed., 6, Baltimore, The Williams & Wilkins Company, 1961, 842 pp.
10. Sections of Neurology and Section of Physiology, Mayo Clinic: Clinical Examinations in Neurology. Ed. 2, Philadelphia, W. B. Saunders Company, 1963, 396 pp.

CHAPTER TEN

THE HIP

ESSENTIAL ANATOMY

The hip is an enarthrodial, spheroidal or ball-and-socket joint formed by the articulation of the rounded head of the femur with the cup-shaped cavity of the acetabulum. It is a weight-bearing joint that combines a wide range of motion with great stability. The hip joint has greater strength and stability but less mobility than the shoulder joint which is also a ball-and-socket joint. Stability of the hip is due to (1) the deep insertion of the head of the femur into the acetabulum, (2) the strong fibrous articular capsule, and (3) the powerful muscles that pass over the joint and insert some distance below the head of the femur thus providing considerable leverage for the femur and stabilization for the joint.

Acetabular Cavity

The acetabular cavity is formed by fusion of the ilium, ischium, and pubis. It is deepest and strongest superiorly and posteriorly where it is subject to the greatest strain when a person is in the erect or stooped position. A mass of fat lies in the fossa at the bottom of the acetabulum. The acetabular cavity is deepened by a circular fibrocartilaginous rim, the glenoid labrum (or cotyloid ligament), that reduces the diameter of the acetabular outlet by forming a tight collar around the head of the femur and thus adds to the stability of the head of the femur in its socket. The lower portion of the labrum is incomplete, forming the acetabular notch. However, a transverse ligament over the acetabular notch completes the fibrous acetabular rim and converts the notch into a foramen through which blood vessels pass into the joint.

Articular Capsule and Ligaments (Fig. 77A)

The hip joint has a strong, dense articular capsule which is attached proximally to the edge of the acetabulum, the glenoid labrum, and the transverse ligament which passes over the acetabular notch. Distally, the capsule surrounds the neck of the femur and is attached anteriorly to the intertrochanteric line and posteriorly to the neck about half an inch above the intertrochanteric crest. Thus all of the anterior surface and the medial half of the posterior surface of the femoral

123

neck are intracapsular. Some of the capsular fibers are reflected upward from their femoral attachment and run along the neck of the femur as longitudinal bands or retinacula. The articular capsule is strong and thick over the upper and anterior portions of the joint; it becomes thinner and relatively weak over the lower and posterior portions of the joint.

The articular capsule is composed of circular and longitudinal fibers. The circular fibers are the deeper ones except over the lower and posterior portions of the capsule where they appear near the surface. The longitudinal fibers are stronger and more numerous than the circular fibers and are divided into distinct bands or accessory ligaments which reinforce the capsule.

Iliofemoral Ligament. This is the strongest and most important of the accessory bands. Crossing the front of the capsule, it extends from the ilium near the anterior inferior spine to the anterior portion of the base of the neck and intertrochanteric line of the femur (Fig. 77A). The lower portion of the iliofemoral ligament divides into two bands, forming an inverted Y shape. It is relaxed in flexion and taut in extension of the thigh and prevents excessive hyperextension of the hip. In the upright position, the iliofemoral ligament keeps the pelvis from rolling backward on the femoral head and stabilizes the hip by pulling the femoral head firmly into its socket.

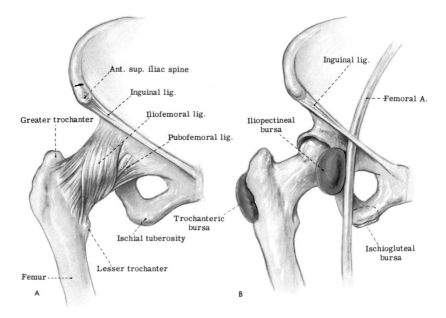

Figure 77. A. Diagram of the anterior aspect of the hip joint and adjacent bony structures. The fibers of the iliofemoral and pubofemoral ligaments fuse with those of the underlying articular capsule. The synovial membrane lines the inner surface of the articular capsule. B. Diagram of the relationship of the iliopectineal, trochanteric, and ischiogluteal bursae to the hip joint and adjacent structures.

124

Pubofemoral and Ischiocapsular Ligaments. These are weaker than the iliofemoral ligament but help reinforce the posterior portion of the capsule. Respectively, they pass obliquely from the pubic and ischial portions of the acetabular rim to the femoral capsular attachment. Throughout their course they blend with the circular fibers of the capsule.

Ligamentum Teres. This is an intracapsular ligament which loosely attaches the femoral head to the lower portion of the acetabulum and adjacent ligaments. It has little effect on the normal motion or stability of the joint but is a channel for blood vessels to the head of the femur.

Iliotibial Band. The iliotibial band is a portion of the fascia lata of the thigh which extends inferiorly from the sacrum, the iliac crest, and the ramus and tuberosity of the ischium over the greater trochanter of the femur and lateral aspect of the thigh to insert into the lateral tuberosity of the tibia, the head of the fibula, the external condyle of the femur, and the entire course of the lateral intermuscular septum existing between the hamstring muscles and the vastus lateralis muscle. The significance of this structure is discussed in the section on "Special Tests for the Hip" on page 141.

Synovial Membrane

The synovial membrane of the hip lines the deep surface of the articular capsule. Proximally, it covers both surfaces of the cartilaginous rim of the acetabulum (glenoid labrum) and a mass of fat in the fossa at the bottom of the acetabulum. The synovial membrane also encloses the ligamentum teres in a sheath of synovial tissue. Distally, the synovial membrane is reflected upward from the femoral attachment of the capsule onto the neck of the femur and extends up to the cartilaginous surface of the femoral head. (Illustration of the synovial membrane of the hip has been omitted because the synovial membrane of the hip is not palpable or visible on physical examination unless a rare synovial cyst of the hip is present.)

Bursae

Figure 77B shows the relationship of the iliopectineal, trochanteric, and ischiogluteal bursae to the joint and adjacent structures.

Iliopectineal Bursa. This bursa lies between the deep surface of the iliopsoas muscle and the anterior surface of the joint. It lies over the anterior portion of the articular capsule between the iliofemoral and pubocapsular ligaments. It communicates with the joint cavity only in about 15 per cent of normal individuals.

125

Trochanteric Bursa. The trochanteric bursa is situated between the gluteus maximus muscle and the posterolateral surface of the greater trochanter. It is a large and usually multilocular bursa but is not palpable or visible unless distended.

Bursae also usually separate the deep surface of the gluteus maximus muscle from the tuberosity of the ischium and from the vastus lateralis muscle.

Ischiogluteal Bursa. The bursa over the ischial tuberosity is known as the "ischiogluteal bursa."

Muscles

Principal Muscles of Motion. The hip joint is surrounded by powerful and well-balanced muscles which not only move the extremity but also help maintain the upright position of the trunk. Extension of the femur on the pelvis is performed by the gluteus maximus, hamstring muscles, and ischial head of the adductor magnus. Flexion of the hip is carried out by the psoas major, iliacus, tensor fasciae latae, rectus femoris, sartorius, pectineus, adductores longus and brevis, and the anterior fibers of the glutei medius and minimus. Abduction is achieved by the glutei medius and minimus, and adduction by the adductores magnus, longus, and brevis, the pectineus, and the gracilis. Rotation of the thigh inward is performed by the gluteus minimus and the anterior fibers of the gluteus medius, the tensor fasciae latae, the adductores longus, brevis, and magnus, the pectineus, and the iliacus and psoas major. Rotation of the thigh outward is effected by the posterior fibers of the gluteus medius, the piriformis, obturatores externus and internus, gemelli superior and inferior, quadratus femoris, gluteus maximus, and the sartorius.

Bony Landmarks

The bony landmarks of the pelvis will be described since the relationship of the pelvis to the femur is important in the evaluation of this joint (Fig. 77A). The crest of the ilium, the ischial tuberosity, and the greater trochanter are readily identifiable landmarks of the bony pelvis and femur. The entire iliac crest, which terminates anteriorly at the anterior superior spine and posteriorly at the posterior superior spine, is palpable subcutaneously.

The ischial tuberosity lies beneath the gluteus maximus and is easily felt when the hip is flexed because the tuberosity is then uncovered by muscle.

The greater trochanter of the femur normally lies the width of the subject's palm below the iliac crest about halfway between the ischial tuberosity and the anterior superior spine. It is located when the subject is in the erect position by finding a flattened depression on the upper lateral aspect of the thigh. In a thin subject the trochanter may produce a prominent projection on the surface of the skin when the hip is abducted and the thigh extended. This results from relaxation of the fascia lata by passive abduction of the thigh, allowing the upper portion of the trochanter to become defined more easily. If the hip is partially flexed and abducted by the examiner, the greater trochanter can be grasped between the fingers and the thumb, and easily outlined.

INSPECTION

Inspection includes evaluation of the patient's gait, functional and actual length of legs and length of thighs, body habitus, nutritional state, spinal curvatures, pelvic tilt, and scars of previous operations or trauma in the region of the hip.

Gait

Normal gait patterns vary widely. In healthy normal gaits the abductor muscles of the weight-bearing extremity contract and hold either both sides of the pelvis level or the side of the pelvis not bearing the weight slightly raised. A "lazy" gait pattern, which is often seen in women, is characterized by sagging of the nonweight-bearing side of the pelvis; an exaggerated swaying motion of the hips results during walking.

Several types of limp or abnormalities of gait are associated with disease of the hip. When the hip is painful or diseased, the body may tilt toward the involved hip and become balanced in this position by leaning to the affected side. This produces an antalgic gait and thrusts the weight of the body directly over the hip joint, decreasing the necessity for contraction of abductor muscles in order to hold the pelvis level and relieving muscle spasm to some extent. If the abductor muscles on the side of the involved hip become weak and are unable to hold the pelvis level when weight is borne on the involved hip, dropping of the pelvis on the side opposite the affected hip may occur and produce a Trendelenburg or abductor limp. The abductor limp causes the upper portion of the body to shift toward the normal side and decreases weight bearing on the involved side. Both of these limps may be caused by a wide variety of lesions, and neither can be considered characteristic of any particular disease. Generally, diseases of the hip that cause pain tend to produce the antalgic limp, whereas diseases which produce an unstable hip and weakness of abductor muscles (such as poliomyelitis or other atrophy of muscles) tend to cause the Trendelenburg or abductor limp. However, either type of limp may be seen in patients with a painful hip or in those with abductor muscle weakness.

Abnormal Positions of the Femur in Relation to the Pelvis

Inspection of the relationship of the femur to the pelvis is of particular importance in the recognition of disease of the hip. Normally, the weight of the body in the upright position is supported equally by both hips and the relationship of the femur to the pelvis is approximately the same on both sides. In the presence of unilateral disease of the hip, the weight of the body in the upright position is often supported mainly on the healthy leg, and in the standing position the leg on the involved side is usually placed in advance of the normal one because of flexion of the involved hip. This may be detected by having the patient stand erect and then alternating the body weight from one leg to the other. One side may be compared with the other by inquiring about the presence or absence of pain and noting disability or muscle spasm on each side in these positions.

Flexion of the Hip. Flexion is one of the most common findings on inspection which suggests abnormality of the hip. The flexed-hip position relaxes the articular capsule of the hip and tends to lessen pain, muscle spasm, and capsular distention. The patient with a flexion deformity of the hip frequently assumes a characteristic position when standing or lying supine on a flat surface. The spinal column is arched anteriorly in the lumbar region with production of lordosis and anterior pelvic tilt. This erroneously appears to reduce the flexion deformity of the hip. When the patient is lying supine on a flat surface, this compensatory pelvic tilt and lordotic curvature of the lumbar portion of the spinal column may allow the thigh to come into contact with the examining table (Fig. 78A). Extension of the flexed hip usually aggravates the pain in the hip by pulling taut the iliofemoral ligament over the anterior portion of the joint and thereby pressing the head of the femur firmly into the acetabulum. Flexion contracture of the hip also is indicated when the patient is lying prone and cannot extend the hip fully or when the examiner cannot lift the thigh into extension without simultaneously lifting the patient's pelvis.

Length of the Legs and Tilting of the Pelvis

Normally, when the patient is in the upright position the anterior-superior iliac spines are level and an imaginary line connecting them forms a right angle with each lower extremity. Apparent changes in the length of the leg may actually be due to lateral tilting of the pelvis associated with abduction or adduction deformities of the hip (see pp.

A.

B.

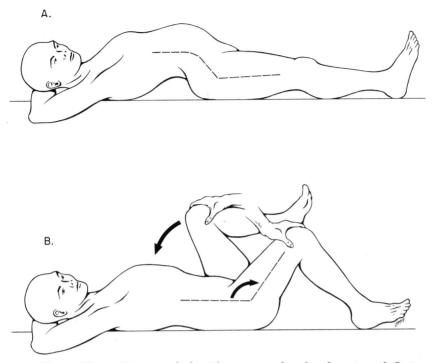

Figure 78.   Diagram of the Thomas test for the detection of flexion deformity of the hip. See text for details. *A.* Flexion deformity of the hip is masked by an abnormal increase in the lumbar lordosis. *B.* Flexion of the opposite hip flattens the lumbar spine and reveals the extent of the flexion deformity in the hip.

105, 136). If because of contractures one leg is in a position of adduction, the lower portion of that leg might cross the opposite normal leg. This position makes walking or weight bearing difficult or impossible. To compensate for this functional impasse, the pelvis is tilted upward on the side of the adducted thigh to help make both legs parallel for standing or walking. Elevation of the pelvis on the side of a fixed adduction deformity pulls the limb upward and makes it appear to be shorter than the other. On actual or bony measurement, however, the lower extremities are equal or as nearly equal as is normal. To restore balance in the upright position and compensate for the apparent (functional) shortness of the leg, the patient may have to stand on the toes of the short leg or flex the knee on the normal side.

     If one hip is held in abduction because of ankylosis or muscle spasm, the leg on the side of the abduction appears to be lengthened in the upright position. This causes an upward tilt of the pelvis on the normal side in an attempt to make the legs more nearly parallel for weight bearing. The actual length of each leg measured from the anterior superior spine of the ilium to the medial malleolus is approximately equal, but measurements from the umbilicus to each medial malleolus would show apparent (functional) lengthening of the leg on the side of abduction.

Asymmetry of the Cutaneous Folds. Asymmetry of the folds of skin in the popliteal or gluteal regions may give information as to the actual length of the leg and the femur when one side is compared to the other. Interpretation of the popliteal and gluteal folds is reliable only when the patient is standing with both legs parallel and both feet positioned firmly on the floor. In the presence of a pelvic tilt, the gluteal skin folds of the buttock will be higher on the side with the elevation of the pelvis than on the opposite side. Thus, if the left leg is actually longer than the right and the patient is standing with both feet on the floor, the gluteal folds on the left will be higher than those on the right. Elevation of the pelvis on the side with a fixed adduction deformity of the hip would also elevate the gluteal folds on the involved side, but the foot on this side would not be firmly on the floor. Asymmetry of the gluteal folds may also result from a gluteal abscess, muscle spasm, posterior dislocation of the hip, and atrophy or hypertrophy of gluteal muscles. When the popliteal creases are level and the patient is standing with both feet on the floor, the tibias and fibulas of the two legs below these creases are of equal length.

Either anterior or posterior dislocation of the hip causes a position of moderate flexion of the knee and hip. Anterior dislocation, however, produces external rotation and abduction of the hip. Posterior dislocation, which is the more common of the two, causes the hip to remain in a position of adduction and internal rotation. Fracture of the femoral neck is associated with acquired external rotation of the involved leg.

PALPATION

Before the examination by palpation is started, it is helpful to have the patient point out areas of pain or tenderness as specifically as possible. The common tendency of patients to do this with the fingers or hand hidden from direct view by the examiner should be avoided by having the patient stand with his or her back or side toward the examiner, or if the patient is being examined in bed, having the patient lie prone. When the muscles adjacent to the hip are relaxed to eliminate the pain of muscle spasm, pain referred from the hip arises from the attachments of the adductor muscles of the hip on the pubis and extends down the anterior and medial aspect of the thigh as far as the knee or arises in the groin in the region of the middle two thirds of the inguinal ligament, in the inferior portion of the buttock, and in the region of the greater trochanter. Sometimes the patient is unable to

130

define the pain as superficial and can locate the area only as "deep" in the general region of the hip. Localization of pain to areas other than these may indicate involvement of structures other than those of the hip even though considered by the patient as occurring in the hip.

After the patient has localized the area of pain or tenderness as specifically as possible, the examiner attempts to define the involved area more accurately by palpation. The following structures are palpated for evidence of soft-tissue swelling, tenderness, and superficial warmth.

Bony Landmarks

These and the method of palpating them have been described in the section on "Anatomy" (see p. 126).

Synovial Membrane

Synovial thickening or distention of the articular capsule from involvement of the hip usually cannot be palpated; rarely a large quantity of synovial fluid may produce palpable swelling and fullness over the anterior portion of the capsule in the region of the iliopectineal bursa if it communicates with the joint and has thereby accumulated some of the fluid. It is difficult to differentiate involvement of the joint from tenderness of the soft-tissue structures overlying it. Occasionally, firm pressure behind and somewhat superior to the greater trochanter may cause the tenderness if synovitis or effusion is present since the synovial membrane is located relatively close to the surface in this area. Localized heat or warmth in the region of the hip usually indicates soft-tissue inflammation rather than disease of the hip because of the deep location of the hip joint.

Disease of the hip, including synovitis, may be suggested by pain in the region of the hip when the patient is supine and relaxed and the examiner percusses the heel with his hand or fist while the patient's leg is extended or when simultaneous firm pressure is applied by the examiner's hands over each greater trochanter. *Percussion of the heel* and *trochanter-to-trochanter pressure* are helpful methods of evaluating involvement of the hip in the patient when examination is limited by the patient's inability to assume an upright position.

Bursae (Fig. 77B)

Iliopectineal Bursa. Fullness and tenderness of this bursa are detected by palpable swelling and tenderness in the area of the middle third of the inguinal ligament and lateral to the femoral pulse. The tenderness is aggravated by extension and reduced or relieved by flexion of the hip. The possibility of a communication between this bursa and the joint (present in 15 per cent of cases) has been mentioned. In this instance extension of the hip increases tension of the fluid in the joint cavity and its communication with the overlying bursa. Thus iliopectineal bursitis may represent either localized bursitis or extension of synovitis of the entire hip through the communication. The latter also is described as a synovial cyst of the hip. The presence or absence of a communication between a synovial cyst of the hip and the iliopectineal bursa usually cannot be determined by physical examination.

Trochanteric Bursa. Trochanteric bursitis causes localized tenderness on palpation in the area of the greater trochanter of the femur. Discrete localization of the tender area by palpation is the most important diagnostic finding of this condition. The pain is usually aggravated by active abduction and rotation of the hip carried out against the resistance of the examiner's counterforce, whereas flexion and extension cause relatively little discomfort. It is difficult to differentiate between a purely bursal reaction and localized tendinitis in the region of the bursa. Since treatment is the same for both conditions, it is not often necessary to establish the difference between these conditions. Careful localization of the tenderness by palpation to the region of the greater trochanter usually is sufficient to differentiate the pain of trochanteric bursitis or tendinitis from referred pain from involvement of the hip.

Ischiogluteal Bursa. Tenderness over the ischial tuberosity may indicate ischiogluteal bursitis ("weavers' bottom") and sometimes is associated with swelling in this region. Tenderness over the ischial tuberosity also may be due to osteitis or inflammation of tendinous attachments.

Other Findings in the Inguinal Region

The inguinal region should be carefully palpated for masses which might result from adenopathy, femoral or inguinal hernia, tumor, aneurysm, or psoas abscess.

MOVEMENT AND RANGE OF MOTION

The hip has a wide range of motion which permits flexion, extension, adduction, abduction, rotation, and circumduction. The angulation between the neck and shaft of the femur partially converts the angular movements of flexion, extension, adduction, and abduction into rotary movements of the femoral head within the acetabulum. When the hip is flexed and abducted, it loses much of the stability observed in the extended position because then only a part of the femoral head is covered by the acetabulum and the remaining portion is covered only by the articular capsule.

Hyperextension

Hyperextension of the hip is measured best while the patient is lying on the abdomen. To prevent the possibility of mistaking motion of the lumbar vertebrae for motion of the hip, the examiner fixes the pelvis and lower vertebrae by applying downward pressure over the sacrum with one hand while the thigh is lifted from the table with the other hand. Normally, hyperextension of the hip of about 15 degrees is possible when the leg and thigh are straight and the pelvis and spinal column are immobilized (Fig. 79). With concurrent motion of the lumbar vertebrae, the hip, and the pelvis, the thigh may be hyperextended to about 40 degrees. Hyperextension is commonly limited in disease of the hip.

Exaggerated lumbar lordosis, if present, must be obliterated in order to determine the actual amount of limitation of extension or flexion deformity in the hip. This can be accomplished by forced flexion of the hip opposite from the one being examined while the patient is lying supine. When this forces the hip on the side being examined into a flexion deformity, the result of the test, known as the Thomas test, is regarded as positive. This finding indicates restriction of extension in the hip (Fig. 78B). The degree of fixed flexion deformity can be estimated by measuring the angle between the involved thigh and the examining table.

Except for hyperextension, motions of the hip are usually best determined with the patient in a supine position.

Flexion

The greatest degree of flexion of the hip is possible when the knee is also flexed. The thigh can be flexed to about 120 degrees from the neutral or extended position (0 or 180 degrees) if the knee has

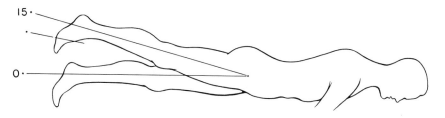

Figure 79. Diagram of normal range of hyperextension of the hip with the pelvis and lumbar veretebrae stabilized. This range is determined with the patient in the prone position.

133

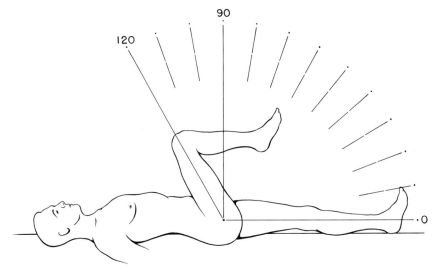

Figure 80.   Range of flexion of the hip with the knee flexed.

been first flexed to about 90 degrees and is held in this position by the examiner. Sometimes the hip can be flexed until the anterior surface of the thigh presses against the anterior abdominal wall (Fig. 80). If the knee cannot be flexed, flexion of the hip can be tested by raising the extended leg off the surface of the table. If the knee remains extended, tension of the hamstring muscles will limit flexion of the hip so that the angle between the thigh and the long axis of the body when the hip is normal may not be more than a right angle (90 degrees; Fig. 81). However, some individuals with apparently normal hips are only able to flex the hip to form an angle of about 75 degrees when the leg is extended, whereas in others the range of motion is much greater than 90 degrees.

Abduction and Adduction

These movements are measured with both thighs and legs in an extended position and parallel to each other while the patient is supine. Measurement is made from the angle formed between an imaginary midline extended from the long axis of the body and the long axis of the leg. The amount of abduction permitted increases with flexion and decreases with extension of the hip. Normally, when the leg and thigh are extended, the hip abducts about 40 to 45 degrees from the neutral position before the pubocapsular and medial portions of the iliofemoral ligaments restrict it. There is, however, considerable variation in the range of abduction beyond 45 degrees in normal individuals (Fig. 82). Limitation of abduction of the hip with the patient lying

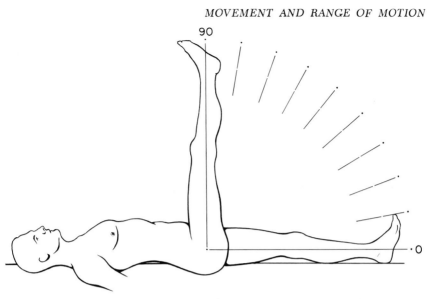

Figure 81. Range of flexion of the hip with the knee extended.

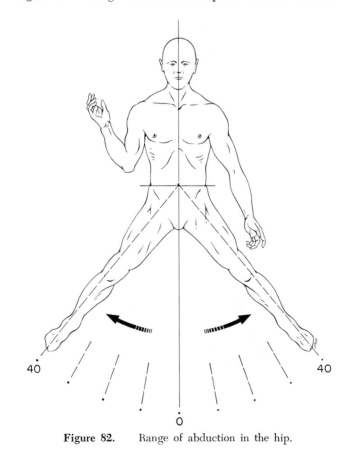

Figure 82. Range of abduction in the hip.

135

flat on his back is the most common limitation of hip motion in the presence of disease of the hip. However, abduction of the hip also may be limited by spasm of the adductor muscles without involvement of the hip.

To test abduction of the hip, the examiner stands at the patient's feet, grasps the patient's extended left leg with the right hand and the patient's extended right leg with the left hand and abducts both hips simultaneously. This allows the examiner to detect minor degrees of limitation of motion by comparing one side with the other. With the patient's legs abducted, the examiner also can detect tilting of the pelvis by first abducting one of the legs and then the other while he observes the patient's pelvis.

Adduction with the leg straight normally is limited by the legs and thighs coming into contact with each other, but adduction with enough flexion of the hip to permit crossing of the legs is usually possible to about 20 to 30 degrees from the neutral (starting) position.

Internal and External Rotation

These movements may be measured while the patient is supine with both the hip and the knee flexed, while the examiner swings the foot inward or medially for measurement of external rotation of the hip and outward or laterally for measurement of internal rotation of the hip (Fig. 83). During this procedure the foot and the thigh are moving in opposite directions. The hip normally rotates inward about 40 degrees and outward about 45 degrees, but the range of rotation varies considerably in normal individuals and both sides should be compared. External rotation is limited by the lateral band of the iliofemoral ligament; internal rotation is limited by the ischiocapsular ligament. Rotation of the hip increases with flexion and decreases with extension of the hip. Limitation of internal rotation of the hip also is one of the earliest and most reliable signs of disease in the hip.

External and internal rotation of the hip can be tested with the patient's hip and knee fully extended while the patient is supine by rolling the thigh, leg, and foot outward and inward.

Rotation of the hip may be tested also when the patient is in the prone position; in this position the thighs and pelvis are well supported by the examining table. With this alternate method the patient's knee is flexed to 90 degrees by raising the foot and leg. The examiner then swings the foot inward for measurement of external rotation of the hip and outward for measurement of internal rotation of the hip while the thigh rests on the examining table (Fig. 84).

A further maneuver which can be used when the examiner wishes to determine whether or not ankylosis is present can be made when the patient is lying supine. The examiner places one hand and forearm

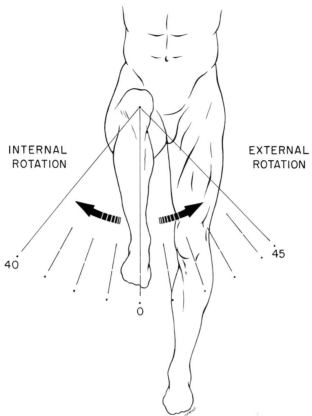

INTERNAL
ROTATION

EXTERNAL
ROTATION

40

45

0

Figure 83. Range of internal and external rotation of the hip with the patient lying supine and with the hip flexed to 90 degrees on the side being examined while the other hip is extended. The examiner swings the foot inward for measurement of external rotation of the hip and outward for measurement of internal rotation of the hip. During this procedure the foot and thigh are moving in opposite directions. See text for details.

under the thigh on the side to be examined, and supports the thigh on his forearm while the other hand is placed on the opposite iliac crest. The thigh is moved gently in various directions. In the presence of ankylosis of the hip the pelvis moves with each movement of the femur.

SPECIAL TESTS FOR THE HIP

Heel-to-Knee Test or Fabere Sign

A simple test for detection of involvement of the hip joint without differentiating the extent of limitation of a specific motion is the heel-to-knee test which involves to some extent several motions of the hip at the same time (Fig. 85). The motions of the hip utilized in this

137

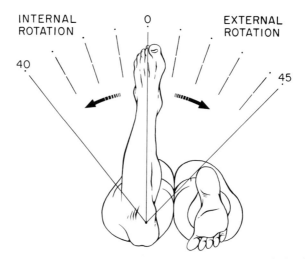

INTERNAL
ROTATION

O

EXTERNAL
ROTATION

40

45

Figure 84. Range of internal and external rotation of the hip with the patient lying prone and with the hip extended to 180 degrees and the knee flexed to 90 degrees on the side being examined while both hip and knee are extended on the opposite side. The examiner swings the foot inward for measurement of external rotation of the hip and outward for measurement of internal rotation of the hip. During this procedure the foot and thigh are moving in opposite directions. See text for details.

test are flexion, abduction, external rotation, and at the completion of the test, extension. The initial letters of these motions were combined by Patrick to designate this test as "fabere sign." (The "f" is sometimes capitalized, but since this is not an eponymic designation, use of the lower-case letter is more appropriate.)

The hip and the knee on the side to be tested are flexed so that the heel lies beside or on top of the opposite extended knee. The hip being examined is then abducted and externally rotated as far as possible. The presence of pain, muscle spasm, or limitation of motion in the region of the hip on the side being examined constitutes a positive result of the test and suggests an abnormality of the hip. When this test gives a negative result, motion is normal and no pain or discomfort occurs, but some patients will describe discomfort in the lumbosacral region of the spinal column, which requires differentiation from the positive response. This test is performed easily and provides a general indication of hip disease but is less reliable for the detection of early disease of the hip than is specific measurement of internal rotation and abduction of the hip.

Measurement of Legs

This is performed most easily with the patient lying supine on a firm, level surface. The legs are extended, are parallel with the long

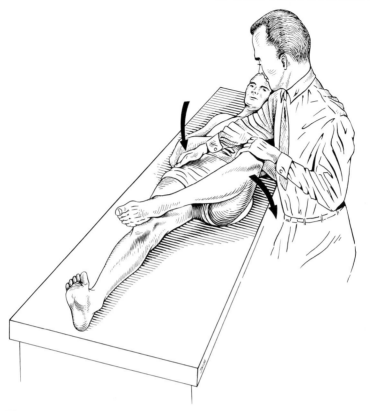

Figure 85.   Heel-to-knee test or fabere sign for the detection of limitation of motion in the hip. See text for details.

axis of the body and are parallel to each other. To prevent lateral tilting of the pelvis, the anterior-superior spines should lie on an imaginary line that is at a right angle to the long axis of the body. When marked scoliosis or severe muscle spasm is present, this may not be possible. The examiner then is alert to the fact that a pelvic tilt produces apparent and not actual shortening of the leg. The length of each leg is measured from the anterior-superior spine to the prominence of the medial malleolus on the same extremity. The measuring tape crosses the anterior surface of the patella at its middle. Comparison of the measurements of the two legs commonly reveals small differences in their length; a difference of less than 1 cm. does not affect the gait. The significance of shortening in one leg as compared to the other is often difficult to evaluate. Shortness of one leg is often asymptomatic.

Shortening of the thigh may be detected by comparing the distances from the anterior superior spine to the distal margin of the medial femoral condyle on the same side. If shortening is present, it may represent shortness or deformity of the femoral head and neck, shortness of the femoral shaft, or dislocation of the femoral head above the acetabulum. If the distances from the prominence of the greater trochanter to the prominence of the lateral femoral condyle are equal in both thighs, the shortening is not in the femoral shaft. An accurate or true measure of the leg length, however, needs to be determined by a scanogram which includes hip, knee, and ankle measured against a scale.

Tests for Congenital Dysplasia or Dislocation of the Hip

This condition may be detected in the following manner in infants: If the infant's hip is flexed to a right angle and then abducted, the lateral aspect of the thigh normally will reach or nearly touch the examining table or the surface on which the patient is lying at the time and will form an angle of almost 180 degrees with the other thigh if both hips are placed in a similar position at the same time. If subluxation of one or both hips is present, abduction is distinctly limited, and the thigh will come only within 45 degrees or less of the examining table. Telescoping or up-and-down (cephalad-caudad) movement of the femur in relation to the pelvis may be demonstrable if the infant's hip is dislocated and the examiner alternately pushes upward and pulls downward on the thigh with the fingers of one hand behind the greater trochanter while the thumb is on the anterior superior iliac spine and the other hand is grasping the patient's knee anteriorly. This maneuver should not be attempted when fracture of the hip is suspected.

Trendelenburg Test

Normally, when a patient bears the weight of the body on one lower extremity, the pelvis on the opposite side may be slightly raised by the contraction of the abductor muscles of the weight-bearing extremity in order to maintain balance. When this function is not normal owing to dislocation of the hip, nonunion of the femoral neck, coxa valga, or marked weakness of the hip abductors, all of the patient's attempts to stand with all the weight of the body on the affected limb cause the pelvis to drop on the opposite side even with full cooperation of the patient because of instability of the hip, lateral displacement of the femur, or lack of a stable fulcrum for the abductor muscles. The Trendelenburg test is positive when the pelvis drops on the side opposite to the weight-bearing extremity (see gait, p. 127). This test is a measure of the patient's ability to use the abductor muscles of the hip properly regardless of whether the patient's habits of walking are good or bad.

Tests for Contraction of the Iliotibial Band

As noted earlier, the iliotibial band is a portion of the fascia lata of the thigh which extends inferiorly from the sacrum, the iliac crest, and the ramus and tuberosity of the ischium over the greater trochanter and lateral aspect of the thigh to insert into the lateral tuberosity of the tibia, the head of the fibula, the external condyle of the femur, and the entire course of the lateral intermuscular septum existing between the hamstring muscles and the vastus lateralis muscle.

The complete deformity resulting from contracture of the iliotibial band consists of flexion, abduction, and external rotation of the hip, genu valgum and flexion contracture of the knee, discrepancy in the length of the lower extremities, external torsion of the tibia on the femur, secondary equinovarus deformity of the foot, external torsion of the femur, obliquity of the pelvis and increased lumbar lordosis. However, since the complete deformity is not always present in patients with contractures of the iliotibial band, the tests described next are helpful in detecting this disorder.

The Abduction or Ober Test. The abduction test for contraction of the iliotibial band is performed with the patient lying on his side. The thigh which is next to the table on which the patient is lying is actively or passively flexed until the lordotic curve of the spine is obliterated. The examiner then places one of his hands on the upper hip in the region of the greater trochanter, grasps the leg on the same (upper) side anteriorly and just below the knee with his other hand, flexes the knee to 90 degrees and fully abducts and hyperextends the thigh. The examiner then slides his hand from its grasping position below the knee down the leg to grasp the ankle anteriorly. Under normal conditions this allows the uppermost thigh to drop in adduction down toward the table. When there is a contraction of the fascia lata or iliotibial band, the uppermost hip remains abducted and the leg does not drop back toward the table. In this situation the iliotibial band can often be palpated easily as a rigid band in the subcutaneous tissues extending between the iliac crest and the anterior portion of the trochanter of the femur.

Adduction or Modified Thomas Test. This is another method for detection of contraction of the iliotibial band. This test is performed with the patient lying supine while the thigh opposite the side to be tested is held in forced flexion against the abdomen in order to stabilize the spinal column. The patient maintains this thigh in forced flexion by clasping his hands together around his leg while the other thigh and leg are tested by being extended or dropped over the end of the examining table and then adducted. If the iliotibial band is contracted, adduction of the extended leg may

141

produce a flexion contracture of the hip when the thigh is perpendicular to the level pelvis. If the flexion contracture of the hip is caused by tightening of the iliotibial band, it can be relieved by abduction of the hip. If the contracted iliotibial band does not produce a significant flexion contracture of the hip, it may also be detected by attempting to adduct the extended leg on the side being examined. If the iliotibial band is contracted, adduction of the extended leg is limited to the extent that it is difficult or impossible to adduct the extended leg across the midline of the body; a partial abduction deformity of the hip is thus revealed by this maneuver. In addition, palpation of the contracted iliotibial band with the hip adducted or in a neutral position gives the feeling of a rigid band in the subcutaneous tissues extending between the iliac crest and the anterior portion of the femoral trochanter.

Suggested Reading for Additional Information

1. Aufranc, O. E.: Constructive Surgery of the Hip. St. Louis, C. V. Mosby Company, 1962, 226 pp.
2. Anson, B. J., and Maddock, W. G.: Callander's Surgical Anatomy. Ed. 4, Philadelphia, W. B. Saunders Company, 1958, pp. 923–949.
3. Hollinshead, W. H.: Anatomy for Surgeons. New York, Paul B. Hoeber, Inc., 1958, vol. 3, pp. 668–685.
4. Turek, S. L.: Orthopaedics: Principles and Their Application. Philadelphia, J. B. Lippincott Company, 1959, pp. 582–636.
5. Johnson, E. W., Jr.: Contractures of the Iliotibial Band. Surg., Gynec. & Obst. 96:599–604 (May) 1953.

CHAPTER ELEVEN

THE KNEE

ESSENTIAL ANATOMY (FIGS. 86 TO 88)

Joint Articular Ligaments and Menisci

The knee is the largest joint in the body. It is a compound condylar joint formed by three articulations which have a common articular cavity. One articulation is located between the lateral femoral and tibial condyles with its corresponding meniscus; another, similarly formed, is situated between the medial femoral and tibial condyles with its corresponding meniscus, and the third lies between the patella and the femur. The fibula does not form part of the knee joint.

The bones of the knee are stabilized by articular ligaments. Ligaments of particular interest are the articular capsule, the ligamentum

143

patellae, the medial (tibial) and lateral (fibular) collateral ligaments, and the anterior and posterior cruciate ligaments. The medial and lateral menisci are fibrocartilaginous disks found within the knee joint interposed between the femoral and tibial condyles.

The *articular capsule* is a thin, fibrous membrane which is strengthened by the fascia lata, tendons, and ligaments surrounding the joint. Anteriorly and superiorly beneath the quadriceps tendon, the articular capsule does not cover the synovial membrane. Posteriorly, however, fibers of the articular capsule enclose the synovial membrane of the suprapatellar pouch and the capsule in this area consists of vertical fibers that arise from the condyles and from the sides of the intercondyloid fossa of the femur. Thus the capsule lies on the side of, and anterior to, the cruciate ligaments which in turn are outside of the joint cavity. Distally, the capsule is connected to the borders of the menisci and then continues to an attachment on the straight margins of each of the tibial condyles.

The *ligamentum patellae* is the extension of the common tendon of the quadriceps which continues from the patella to the tibial tuberosity. A small, triangular fat pad, known as the infrapatellar fat pad, lies below the patella between the ligamentum patellae and the synovial membrane (Fig. 86).

The *collateral ligaments* lend lateral and medial support to the joint. The lateral collateral ligament is a strong, rounded, fibrous cord attached superiorly to the lateral femoral condyle and inferiorly to the lateral side of the fibular head. The medial collateral ligament is a broad, flat, membranous band attached proximally to the medial condyle of the femur just below the adductor tubercle, and distally to the medial condyle of the tibia and to the medial surface of the tibia.

The two *cruciate ligaments* give support in the anteroposterior plane. The anterior (medial) cruciate ligament is attached anteriorly to the intercondyloid eminence of the tibia and extends posteriorly and superiorly to the lateral femoral condyle on its medial and posterior portion. The posterior (lateral) cruciate ligament is attached to the posterior intercondyloid fossa of the tibia and to the posterior portion of the lateral meniscus. It passes superiorly and anteriorly to the medial femoral condyle on its lateral and anterior portion. The synovial membrane covers a large portion of the cruciate ligaments, which, therefore, are situated anatomically outside the synovial cavity.

The *medial and lateral menisci* are wedge-shaped, crescentic, fibrocartilaginous disks. The outside edge of each meniscus is thick and is attached to the articular capsule. The inside edge is thin and unattached. The inferior surfaces are flat and rest on the flat surface of the head of the tibia. The superior surfaces are concave and conform to the surfaces of the femoral condyles with which they come in contact.

144

Synovial Membrane and Adjacent Bursae

The synovial membrane of the knee is the largest in the body (Fig. 86). At the superior border of the patella, it forms a sac or pouch beneath the quadriceps femoris muscle on the anterior aspect of the femur. The suprapatellar reflection of the synovial membrane of the knee begins embryonically as a separate bursa; however, in most cases it communicates freely with the articular synovial space. Thus it is appropriate to recognize this synovial reflection as the suprapatellar reflection or pouch of the knee rather than as a suprapatellar bursa. The superior reflection of the suprapatellar pouch normally extends as much as 6 cm. above the superior pole of the patella.

On each side of the patella, the synovial membrane of the knee extends under the aponeuroses of the vastus medialis and vastus lateralis muscles which are part of the quadriceps femoris group of muscles, being somewhat more extensive on the medial aspect of the patella.

The region of the knee contains numerous bursae. Only the most constant and significant of these will be described (Figs. 86 to 88).

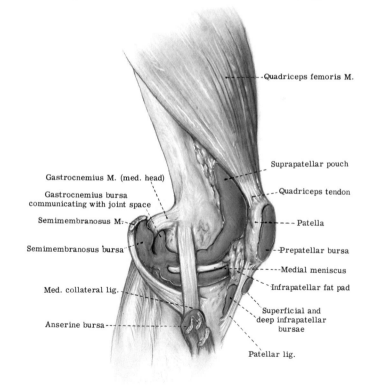

Figure 86. Medial aspect of knee showing distribution of synovial membrane and adjacent bursae when distended.

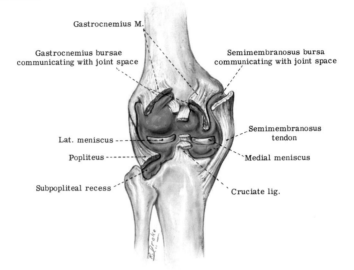

Figure 87.   Posterior aspect of knee joint showing distribution of synovial membrane and adjacent bursae when distended.

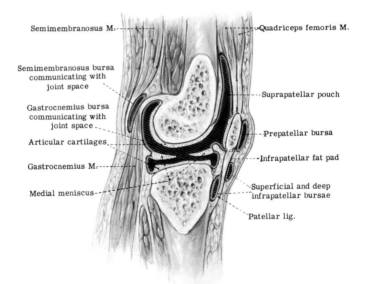

Figure 88.   Schematic sagittal section of knee through area medial to midline showing relationship of synovial membrane and adjacent bursae to other joint structures.

A relatively large *prepatellar bursa* lies on the anterior aspect of the knee and separates the skin from the patella. A small *superficial infrapatellar bursa* is located between the skin and the proximal portion of the ligamentum patellae and a deep *infrapatellar bursa* lies beneath the distal portion of the ligamentum patellae. Posteriorly the *subpopliteal recess* is located on the lateral aspect of the joint and separates the

146

tendon of the popliteus muscle from the lateral condyle of the femur; it is usually an extension from the synovial membrane of the knee joint. A *gastrocnemius bursa* lies on the posterior and lateral aspects of the joint between the lateral head of the gastrocnemius muscle and the articular capsule and usually communicates with the knee joint. *Another gastrocnemius bursa* is situated on the posterior and medial aspects of the joint between the medial head of the gastrocnemius muscle and the articular capsule; this bursa also usually communicates with the knee joint and with the semimembranosus bursa which lies superficial to it. The rather large *semimembranosus bursa* is located posteriorly on the medial aspect of the knee. It lies between the semimembranosus and the medial head of the gastrocnemius. The *anserine bursa* is located on the medial aspect of the knee and lies between the medial collateral ligament and the tendons of the sartorius, gracilis, and semitendinosus muscles.

Muscles

Among the muscles which move and lend support to the knee, the *quadriceps femoris* is of particular importance. This muscle is the great extensor muscle of the leg and covers the anterior and lateral portions of the thigh. It has four heads which merge into a common tendon. The lateral portion is the vastus lateralis, and the medial portion is the vastus medialis. Between them are the vastus intermedius and the rectus femoris, the former lying beneath the latter. The common tendon of the quadriceps femoris continues distally to enclose the patella, the largest sesamoid bone in the body, as it passes over the knee joint to merge with the ligamentum patellae and inserts into the tibial tuberosity. Flexion of the leg on the thigh is performed mainly by the *hamstring muscles* (biceps femoris, semitendinosus, and semimembranosus) which are situated on the posterior aspect of the thigh. External rotation of the tibia and fibula on the femoral condyles is accomplished by the biceps femoris. Internal rotation of the tibia and fibula on the femoral condyles is accomplished primarily by the popliteus and semitendinosus muscles. The *gastrocnemius muscle* which forms a large portion of the calf helps to limit hyperextension of the knee and also plantar flexes the foot.

INSPECTION

The knees should be observed for evidence of deformity or instability both with and without weight bearing. Knees may be angulated. When lateral angulation occurs, the condition is called "genu varum" (bowlegs; Fig. 89); when angulation is medial, the condition is called "genu valgum" (knock knees; Fig. 90). Backward bowling of the knee, genu recurvatum, results from hyperextension of the joint. An angulation anteriorly is described as a flexion contracture of the knee or as limitation

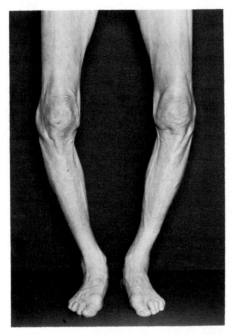

Figure 89. Marked instability and genu varum (bowlegs) of both knees in a patient with degenerative disease of the knees.

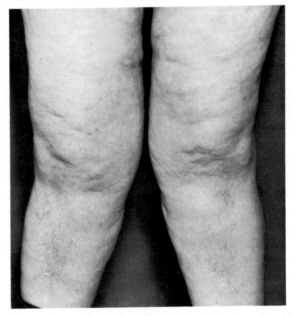

Figure 90. Genu valgum (knock knees) and degenerative disease of both knees.

of full extension of the knee. Observation of the range of motion and the manner in which the joint is used during ambulation also may reveal a limp, hypermobility, contracture, sudden locking, or sudden buckling (giving way) of the knee.

The knees generally are inspected best with the patient relaxed and supine and with the knees extended as fully as possible. A normal knee has distinct landmarks with concavities on each side of, and superior to, the patella. These depressions tend to disappear, and outward bulging may even occur in the presence of synovial thickening or effusion (Fig. 91). Sometimes synovial effusion in the knee may be detected by compressing the suprapatellar pouch with one hand as will be described in the section on "Palpation" and by carefully observing the concave or shallow areas of the joint capsule as they become distended and bulge medially and laterally between the patella and the tibiofemoral margins (see Fig. 104). Release of the pressure on the suprapatellar pouch may cause distention of the articular capsule to disappear if synovial effusion is present. When the synovial membrane and articular capsule are distended by fluid, the knee may be held in a position of 15 to 20 degrees of flexion since this position provides the synovial cavity with its maximal capacity to hold fluid and causes less discomfort from distention than any other position.

Synovitis of the knee is most obvious on inspection by the distention and swelling of the suprapatellar pouch. In such cases inspection may disclose abnormal fullness in the distal anterior portion of the

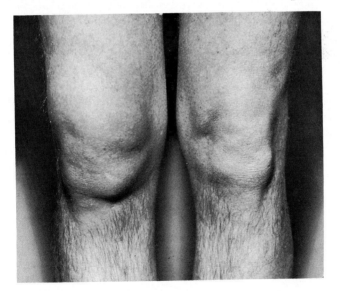

Figure 91. Mild synovitis (grade 1+) of right knee showing loss of normal contours and mild distention and fullness of suprapatellar pouch in a patient with rheumatoid arthritis. Note normal landmarks on left knee with depressed areas on each side of patella.

149

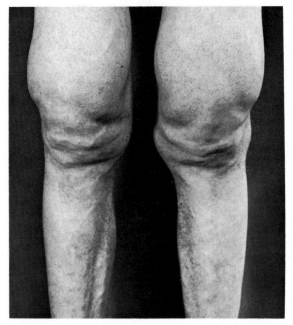

Figure 92.   Marked synovitis (grade 4) of both knees of a patient with rheumatoid arthritis. Extensive fullness and swelling of the suprapatellar pouch are evident.

thigh, which is often even more readily noticeable than the absence of the normal depressed contours adjacent to the patella. This fullness or swelling commonly extends about 5 to 6 cm. above the superior border of the patella, conforming to the extent of the anatomic reflection of this portion of the synovial membrane (Figs. 91 and 92).

Abnormal swelling in other locations adjacent to the knee should be differentiated from synovial thickening or effusion or both. If the *prepatellar bursa* becomes distended, swelling develops on the anterior aspect of the knee between the patella and the overlying skin. Sharply demarcated margins usually indicate that the swelling is localized to the bursa and is not within the distribution of the synovial membrane of the knee. The skin overlying the prepatellar bursa may be shiny, atrophic, reddened, coarse, or thick (Figs. 93 and 94).

Cystic *swellings of the menisci* may occur and typically are localized to the medial or lateral regions of the joint space; such cysts arise more commonly on the lateral than on the medial aspect of the joint and are noted most readily with the knee flexed.

Swelling in the region of the popliteal space may be caused by distention of the semimembranosus bursa, the medial or lateral gastrocnemius bursa, or by posterior herniation of the articular capsule and synovial membrane (Fig. 87). Distention of these structures produces a synovial-lined *popliteal* (*"Baker's"*) *cyst* which usually is an extension

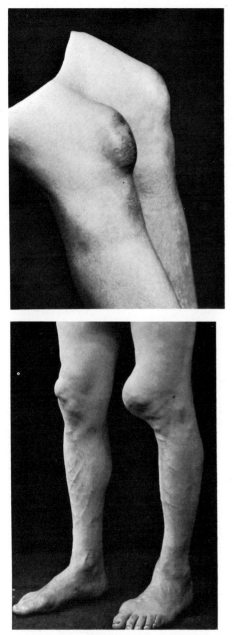

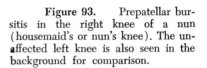

Figure 93. Prepatellar bursitis in the right knee of a nun (housemaid's or nun's knee). The un-affected left knee is also seen in the background for comparison.

Figure 94. Tophaceous gout involving both knees with marked prepatellar bursitis on the left and mild prepatellar bursitis on the right. There is no evidence of synovitis in either knee.

of the synovial membrane of the knee joint (see p. 161). Distention of the semimembranosus bursa, which is situated posteriorly on the medial side of the knee, causes an ovoid swelling on the medial side of the popliteal space.

A popliteal cyst is usually more prominent with the knee extended and tends to become less tense and less prominent with the knee flexed. Flexion of the knee may be restricted by a popliteal cyst. Occasionally

151

a popliteal cyst may dissect downward into the calf muscles and produce an increased diameter and abnormal fullness of the middle or lower part of the leg (Fig. 95). Sometimes a popliteal cyst alone or its extension into the muscles of the calf may obstruct the veins or lymph vessels and cause swelling and dependent edema in the involved leg (Fig. 96). If the dissection or extension of the cyst occurs acutely, localized

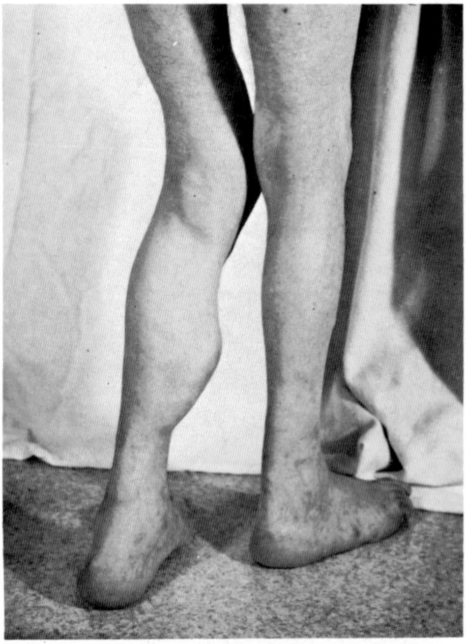

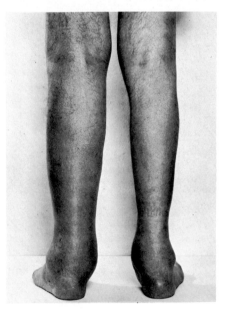

Figure 95.   Extension of a popliteal cyst into the left leg of a patient with rheumatoid arthritis, producing a bulge in the inferior and medial aspect of the calf.

Figure 96.   Popliteal cyst with secondary lymphedema of the left leg in a patient with rheumatoid arthritis. The cyst extends almost 18 cm. into the muscles of the calf.

heat or redness, pain, and swelling may appear, and it may be necessary to distinguish the condition from phlebitis.

The anterior aspect of both thighs should be observed carefully for evidence of atrophy of the quadriceps femoris muscle. Atrophy in this muscle is a particularly significant finding since the quadriceps femoris is the great extensor muscle of the knee and is essential for maintaining stability of this joint on weight bearing. Atrophy of the quadriceps femoris commonly occurs in chronic disorders or with disuse of the knee. The medial (vastus medialis) portion of the quadriceps usually atrophies earliest; this change is easily overlooked since this portion of the quadriceps is relatively small. The vastus medialis is responsible for the final 10 degrees of extension of the knee and without its use the patient cannot maintain the knee in a completely extended position against gravity, nor can he walk with the knee straightened out unless the knee is locked in a position of maximal extension or hyperextension. Although atrophy of the quadriceps makes synovial effusion more evident, it also may give a misleading impression of the amount of enlargement of the knee (Figs. 97 and 98).

When it occurs, dislocation of the patella is seen on full extension of the knee and occurs laterally.

PALPATION

Whenever possible, it is advantageous to palpate the knee with the patient supine and the knee in as complete extension as possible.

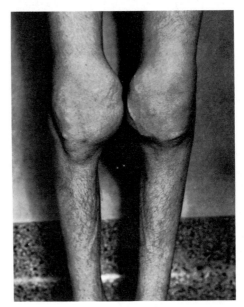

Figure 97. Marked synovitis of both knees (grade 3 on right and grade 2+ on left) of a patient with arthritis and chronic ulcerative colitis. More than the usual degree of medial pouching of the articular capsule and synovial membrane is evident as is considerable atrophy of the quadriceps femoris and other muscles of the leg.

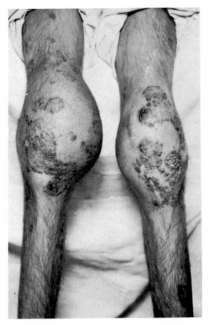

Figure 98.   Psoriatic arthritis with extensive synovitis in both knees (grade 3 on right and grade 2— on left) and marked atrophy of muscles in the thighs and legs. The atrophy of the muscles creates an impression of exaggerated enlargement of the knees.

If the quadriceps femoris muscle is not adequately relaxed, slight abnormalities in the underlying suprapatellar pouch or other portions of the synovial reflection cannot be palpated satisfactorily. Occasionally the examiner may prefer to palpate the knee when the patient is in a sitting position with the leg extended or the knee flexed a few degrees. For some patients this position may result in more relaxation of the leg and thigh muscles than is accomplished in the supine position. However, in this chapter, examination of each knee will be described from the patient's right side with the patient supine.

Synovial Membrane

Synovitis.   For palpation of the suprapatellar pouch, the patient's hips should be abducted enough to prevent contact of the knees, and the knees should be relaxed and fully extended. The examiner places his left hand lightly on the anterior aspect of the thigh about 10 cm. above the superior border of the patella. The thumb is placed medially and the fingers are located laterally (for the left thigh) in a position that might be used to grasp the quadriceps muscle (Fig. 99). With the thumb and fingers exerting light to mild pressure, the examiner carefully palpates the underlying tissues as the hand is moved gradually toward the knee joint in an attempt to locate the superior edge of the synovial reflection of the suprapatellar pouch. The medial and lateral aspects of the quadriceps are palpated for swelling. As the soft tissues in this region are palpated under the fingers, the consistency, nodularity, thickness, warmth, and tenderness of the skin, subcutaneous tissue, and muscles are noted. If excess fluid is present, it is often helpful if the examiner's right hand is used to push superiorly any synovial fluid from the lower recesses of the synovial cavity to distend the suprapatellar pouch more and make it more easily palpable.

When a soft-tissue swelling with a somewhat different consistency from that of normal muscles and other soft tissues is palpated less than 10 cm. above the knee as just described, synovitis of the supra-patellar pouch is recognized. The swelling of synovitis seems fluctuant or "boggy" in comparison with the more solid consistency of muscles and adjacent soft tissues. The medial border of the suprapatellar pouch is particularly likely to be palpable since it lies under the vastus medialis muscle, the first portion of the quadriceps femoris to become atrophied. Distention or thickening of the suprapatellar pouch may be caused by synovial thickening, synovial effusion, and tumors; areas of nodularity and induration alone or in combination may be caused by fibrin masses, loose bodies, reaction from previous steroid or other intra-articular injections, and rarely in present-day clinical experience, tuberculoma. Since the suprapatellar pouch lies relatively close to the surface, the discovery of localized warmth and tenderness in this area also helps in the detection of significant inflammation of the synovial membrane.

In the next maneuver the examiner places his left hand just above the patella to compress the suprapatellar pouch firmly (Fig. 100). Compression of the suprapatella pouch tends to force synovial fluid from

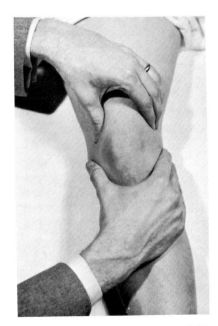

Figure 99. Palpation of the suprapatellar synovial pouch of the left knee. The examiner is standing on the patient's right side. The examiner's right hand firmly slides up from below and compresses the inferior portions of the synovial cavity. The right thumb and forefinger are over the medial and lateral joint spaces, respectively. The left thumb and fingers are palpating the lateral and medial borders of the suprapatellar synovial pouch. See text for details.

155

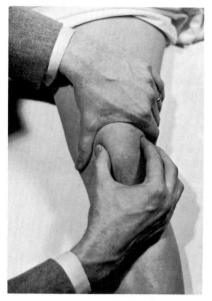

Figure 100.   Palpation of the synovial membrane of the left knee. The examiner's left hand is compressing the suprapatellar pouch. The right thumb and forefinger are lightly palpating the space between the patella and joint proper for evidence of fluctuant distention. See text for details.

the pouch into the inferior portions of the articular synovial cavity. As a result the synovial membrane distends and is more easily palpable in regions adjacent to the articular cavity. While the examiner's left hand maintains pressure over the suprapatellar pouch, he places the right thumb medially and the fingers of the right hand laterally (for the left thigh and leg) between the patella and the tibiofemoral joint. This area is then palpated between the examining thumb and fingers for evidence of abnormal soft-tissue swelling or fluctuant distention of the articular capsule and synovial membrane. Care should be taken not to push the patella, fat pads, and adjacent soft tissues inferiorly or distally with the left hand since this may produce a misleading impression of abnormal soft-tissue swelling in the area being palpated by the fingers and thumb of the right hand. Thickening or distention of the synovial membrane is palpated most easily on the medial aspect of the knee between the patella and the region of the tibiofemoral joint space; normally the synovial membrane is not palpable in this area. A thickened synovial membrane has a "doughy" or "boggy" consistency and also may be fluctuant and accentuated if excessive synovial fluid is present.

Sometimes the margins of the synovial reflection can be palpated over the tibiofemoral joint space on the medial aspect of the knee just distal to the level of the midportion of the patella. The area for palpation of the synovial membrane over the region of the joint space is relatively small; therefore, more experience is required to demonstrate synovitis here than in the suprapatellar area. Some rheumatologists consider the area over the tibiofemoral joint space on the medial aspect of the knee the most reliable site for the detection of mild synovitis and the differentiation of thickening and effusion of the knee joint. The articular capsule and synovial membrane can be palpated particularly well in this area because the overlying tissues are thin and the synovial membrane can be palpated against the adjacent bony structures. While the examiner's left hand is maintaining pressure over the suprapatellar pouch, the right hand in the same finger-thumb position as before is moved toward the articular space from a starting point about 5 cm. distal to the inferior border of the patella. Again care should be taken to avoid pushing suprapatellar and infrapatellar soft tissues and fat pads distally when the suprapatellar pouch is being compressed, since these displaced tissues when palpated by the fingers of the right hand may give a misleading impression of synovitis. As the right hand is moved upward, the thumb and fingers soon come to the tibiofemoral joint space which is palpable in the supine position as an almost vertical groove along the medial and lateral aspect of the knee. (See Figure 101 for positioning of the right thumb and forefinger over the medial and lateral aspects of the joint space, respectively.) If the synovial membrane is thickened or distended, the edges of the synovial membrane can be delineated over the region of the joint space and adjacent bony structures. Abnormalities of the synovial membrane are usually felt more easily over the medial than over the lateral aspect of the joint space. The soft-tissue swelling of synovitis characteristically fans out sharply on the medial aspect of the knee with its apex facing posteriorly toward the joint space.

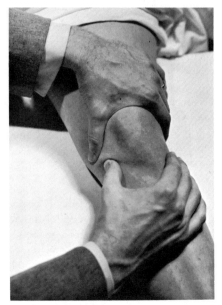

Figure 101. Palpation for synovial thickening and effusion over the medial aspect of the joint space of the left knee. The right thumb is palpating the medial part of the joint space. The left hand alternately applies and releases pressure on the suprapatellar pouch so that the right thumb on the joint space may detect any changes in synovial distention. See text for details.

157

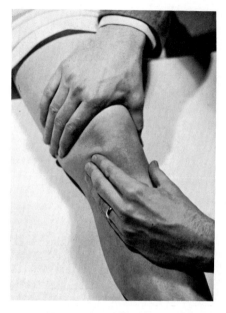

Figure 102. Palpation for synovial thickening and effusion over the medial aspect of the left knee using an alternate method of examination. The examiner is now on the patient's left side so that the left hand is comfortable while the fingers of the left hand carefully palpate the medial aspect of the joint space. The right hand alternately applies and releases pressure on the suprapatellar pouch. The fingers over the joint space may detect changes in synovial distention during this maneuver.

Figure 102 shows an alternate method of palpation for synovitis. The right hand compresses the suprapatellar pouch and the fingers of the left hand palpate the medial joint space.

Since the synovial fluid lies in a closed sac, compressing the fluid in the extreme limits of the synovial reflection over the region of the joint space, as described, causes the edge of the synovial membrane to become palpable as a bulge, which represents both the membrane and the movable fluid within the joint cavity. If this bulge disappears following release of compression on the suprapatellar pouch, the palpable distention may be considered to have represented a synovial effusion; whereas, if it persists, it may be indicative of a thickened synovial membrane. Reliable differentiation between synovial thickening and articular effusion, however, is not always possible by the physical examination. Usually palpation is performed simultaneously for effusion and synovial thickening, and frequently both effusion and synovial thickening are present in the same joint.

Ballottement of the Patella. This may be possible when effusion is present, but it requires a relatively large amount of joint fluid and is not a sensitive method for the detection of a small quantity of fluid in the knee. To perform ballottement of the patella, the examiner compresses the suprapatellar pouch with his left hand and ballots the patella against the femur in an anteroposterior direction with the forefinger of his right hand (Fig. 103).

Bulge Sign. Another maneuver which is most useful for the detection of minor degrees of effusion is referred to as the "bulge sign." For this examination the knee is extended fully while the patient is

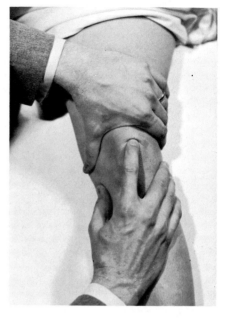

Figure 103. Palpation for effusion by ballottement of the patella of the left knee. The left hand is compressing the suprapatellar pouch. The right forefinger is ballotting the patella in an anteroposterior direction.

in a horizontal resting position with the muscles relaxed. The medial aspect of the knee is stroked and pressure is applied cephalad with one hand by the examiner to express the synovial fluid from this area. The examiner then taps the lateral aspect of the knee with the other hand. A distinct fluid wave or bulge will appear soon afterward on the medial aspect of the knee between the patella and the femur if even a little fluid is present. It may be necessary to tap in several areas on the lateral aspect of the knee to localize the region which produces the maximal fluid wave, but the lateral aspect of the knee just above the midportion of the patella usually is the most effective site. Often this area can be localized so that pressure with only one or two fingertips causes a distinctly visible bulge on the medial aspect of the knee (Fig. 104). A reversal of this technic, accomplished by stroking the lateral aspect of the knee and tapping over the medial aspect, usually produces the same type of bulge, but synovial fluid may be less easily demonstrated than by stroking over the medial aspect and tapping over the lateral aspect. This maneuver reveals effusion of minor degrees that often cannot be detected by other methods and is most reliable when only a small amount of joint fluid is present (4 to 8 ml.) and the synovial membrane is not detectably thickened. This maneuver has been attributed on some occasions to E. G. L. Bywaters, J. H. Kellgren, or Paul Wood, but each has disclaimed originating this test in favor of a previous unknown observer of this phenomenon. Thus, the term "bulge sign" has been used as a convenient and anonymous descriptive indication of this physical finding.

159

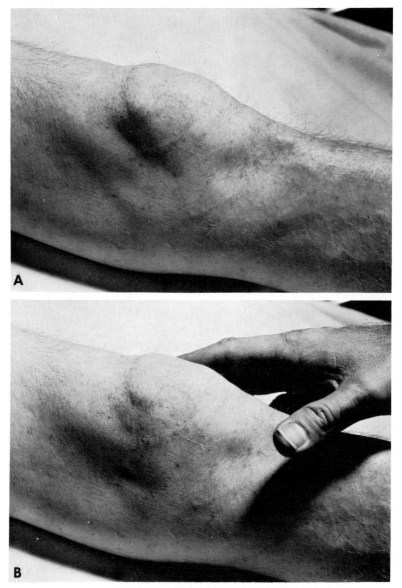

Figure 104.   Bulge sign for demonstration of small synovial effusions of the knee. *A.* View of left knee from medial aspect showing depressed (shaded) area after this area has been stroked as described in the text to move the synovial fluid out of this area. *B.* Same view showing bulge in the depressed area seen in *A* created by tapping lateral aspect of knee to move the synovial fluid back into the medial aspect of knee.

160

Popliteal Space

The posterior aspect of the knee is palpated for evidence of a fluctuant synovial outpouching or cyst in the popliteal space. A synovial cyst in this area is also known as "Baker's cyst" (see p. 150). When the lesion is sufficiently large, its cystic nature may be recognized by transillumination of the involved area.

A popliteal cyst almost always communicates with the synovial cavity of the knee and may fluctuate in size as fluid moves in and out of the joint cavity if the communication between the cyst and joint cavity remains unobstructed. When the opening is very small (often 1 mm. or less in diameter) or when the contents of the cyst are in a semisolid state and mucofibrin or rice bodies are present, a communication may not be demonstrable. Frequently the cyst is most prominent and tense when the knee is extended and tends to be least prominent when the knee is flexed. It is advisable, however, to palpate the popliteal space in both positions. Compression of the suprapatellar pouch may further distend a popliteal cyst to the point where it is easily outlined. The cyst may be tender or warm on palpation if the synovitis has resulted from inflammatory processes and is sufficiently severe to produce such cutaneous reactions.

Examination of the leg may reveal fluctuant fullness, warmth, tenderness, redness, or an increased diameter of the calf if a popliteal cyst has dissected into the posterior or posteromedial aspect of the leg. Rarely the dissection may extend as far as the Achilles tendon. Pressure on the suprapatellar pouch followed by an accompanying pressure on the popliteal space may cause distention of a cystic synovial extension in the leg so that the cystic lesion bulges or points in the region of the calf. It is often helpful to observe and palpate a popliteal cyst or its extension into the calf with the patient standing in order to localize the lesion more accurately.

Popliteal cysts when localized to the popliteal space also must be differentiated from fat pads, aneurysms, neoplasms, localized infections, and varicosities.

Tibial and Femoral Articular Margins

The margins of the bones should be palpated for articular bony lipping or exostosis. Such spurs are palpable as irregular bony edges and often can be felt along the tibial or femoral margins of the knee joint.

Bursae

The prepatellar bursa is easily palpable when distended, but certain other bursae in the region of the knee (for example, the anserine,

161

the superficial and the deep infrapatellar) are smaller and more difficult to recognize by palpation even when tender or enlarged (Figs. 86 and 88). By localizing palpable swelling and tenderness to the region of the bursa rather than to the distribution of the synovial membrane, the examiner can differentiate bursal involvement from that of the articular synovial membrane. Thus the reaction of anserine bursitis is restricted to the medial aspect of the knee and lies between the medial collateral ligament and the tendons of the sartorius, gracilis, and semitendinous muscles. Prepatellar bursitis (housemaid's or nun's knee) is characterized by swelling and tenderness of the bursa which raises the skin over the anterior aspect of patella (Fig. 93). When the bursa is markedly enlarged, prepatellar bursitis can simulate articular synovitis unless the bursal margins are carefully delineated by palpation. Both the bursal and synovial linings may be affected simultaneously, but by careful palpation the involvement of each may be distinguished from that of the other.

Infrapatellar Fat Pad

The infrapatellar fat pad lies beneath the patellar ligament, but when it is distended, it is usually palpable as a soft-tissue fullness and tenderness overlying the patellar ligament and to either side of it (Figs. 86 and 88). Tenderness of the fat pad usually can be differentiated from involvement of adjacent structures by localization of tenderness and swelling to the region of the fat pad.

Patella

Palpation of the patella may reveal several abnormalities. The patella is first palpated with the knee extended in a horizontal position and with the quadriceps femoris relaxed. The patella is pushed firmly downward against the femur by one hand of the examiner and then is moved about so that the articular surface of each quadrant of the patella comes into contact with the femur. Pain or tenderness or grating on rubbing the patella against the femur results from damage to the patellofemoral surfaces.

Crepitus or grating sensation may be felt over the patella by the examiner when he holds his hand on the patella while the knee is flexed and extended either actively or passively or when the patella is moved while the knee is held by the examiner in either the extended or semiflexed position. Although patellofemoral crepitus is often associated with degenerative diseases of the knee or chondromalacia of the patella, crepitus is often misleading and is of relatively little diagnostic value unless it is pronounced since it is not uncommonly found in otherwise asymptomatic knees.

162

If grating sensations and tenderness noted during active flexion and extension of the knee are caused by abnormalities of the patello-femoral surfaces, these signs may disappear when the knee is moved passively by the examiner with the patella held away from the femur. This maneuver is helpful in differentiating chondromalacia of the patella from changes in the tibiofemoral joint, for in the latter instance the grating or tenderness persists.

Palpation of the undersurface of the patella may reveal tenderness if chondromalacia is present. To palpate the undersurface of the patella, the patella is displaced first to one side and then to the other. The amount of displacement possible varies considerably from one individual to another. Frequently only the median ridge of the undersurface of the patella can be felt. When tenderness is present both on grating the patella against the femur and on palpation of the undersurface of the median margin of the patella, it is of significance if it is persistent and present in the same portion of the patella.

Menisci and Collateral Ligaments

Tenderness localized to the medial or lateral aspect of the joint space between the tibia and the femur and below the femoral condyles suggests a tear or some other disorder of the meniscus. The medial meniscus is involved in tears or degenerative changes more frequently than is the lateral meniscus. In contrast, tenderness along the ligamentous attachments over the medial or lateral femoral condyles extending above the region of the joint space suggests a disorder of the collateral ligaments. The medial collateral ligament is involved more frequently than the lateral ligament.

Lesions of the collateral ligaments may be differentiated from those of the menisci by abduction and adduction of the tibia with the femur stabilized.

Abduction Test. This test consists of a valgus strain applied to the lateral aspect of the knee joint by the examiner. The patient should be supine. The examiner firmly grasps the lower part of the patient's thigh on the anterolateral aspect to fix the lower end of the femur and thus prevent abduction of the femur. The examiner also can create a fulcrum to stabilize the patient's femur by pressing his fully flexed knee against the lower lateral aspect of the patient's thigh. After stabilizing the femur and while the patient's knee is in complete extension, the examiner abducts the tibia with one hand by pulling the distal end of the patient's leg outward. This maneuver tends to expand the medial aspect of the tibiofemoral joint, lessening pressure on the medial meniscus and compressing the lateral meniscus of the knee. When this produces pain on the lateral aspect of the knee, it usually indicates that the pain arises from the lateral meniscus. The

163

same maneuver relaxes the lateral collateral ligament and tenses the medial collateral ligament. Thus, if the pain is on the medial aspect of the knee, it is usually due to the strain on the medial collateral ligament. Digital palpation with the examiner's other hand often can localize the area of maximal tenderness as being near the medial femoral condyle rather than on the joint.

Adduction Test. This consists of applying a varus strain to the medial aspect of the knee joint by using the examiner's hand or knee as a fulcrum as described for the abduction test, except that in this instance the pressure or stabilization is applied to the femur from the medial side of the knee being tested. The examiner stabilizes the patient's femur with his knee while he adducts the tibia by pulling the distal end of the patient's leg inward. This tends to open the lateral aspect of the tibiofemoral joint and to compress the medial aspect. This maneuver produces pain on the lateral aspect of the knee because of ligamentous stretching, if there is a lesion in the lateral collateral ligament; sometimes the point of maximal tenderness can be localized by palpation to the area adjacent to the lateral femoral condyle rather than over the joint space. This maneuver also may cause pain on the medial aspect of the joint because of compression if there is a lesion in the medial meniscus. Thus while either the abduction or adduction test may produce pain in the presence of a disorder of a meniscus or collateral ligament, careful localization of the pain will often enable the examiner to differentiate a lesion of the meniscus from a disorder of the collateral ligament; however, these tests are of more value in excluding a disorder of the collateral ligament than in excluding a tear in the meniscus.

Other Maneuvers or Tests. A variation of the abduction and adduction maneuvers can be performed by having the patient stand with his foot inverted and by placing a lift of solid material such as boards, books or magazines about 2.5 to 4.0 cm. in thickness under the medial side of the heel and sole. This increases the mechanical intra-articular pressure on the medial side of the knee in the region of the meniscus and also increases the tendinous pull extra-articularly on the lateral side of the knee to a lesser extent. With the patient standing on an everted foot, the reverse is accomplished.

Sometimes evidence of a tear in the posterior portion of either meniscus can be obtained as follows: The knee is fully flexed while the examiner places one hand over the anterior aspect of the knee with the index finger flattened along the line of the joint on one side and with the thumb on the other. Medial and lateral rotatory movements of the tibia are performed with the examiner's other hand while the knee is moved from full flexion to extension by the examiner. This maneuver, known as McMurray's sign, will often produce a palpable and sometimes audible snapping when the torn meniscus moves in and out of place. It may

164

cause transient pain. A sudden click may be felt during active extension of the knee when the lateral meniscus is torn.

Cysts of the menisci may produce localized swelling and tenderness in the region of the joint space which is palpable between the tibial and femoral condyles medially or laterally as described. These cysts usually arise on the lateral aspect of the joint and are noticed most easily when the knee is flexed.

MOVEMENT AND RANGE OF MOTION

The knee should normally extend to a straight line (0 or 180 degrees) and frequently can be hyperextended up to 15 degrees. The degree of extension is determined by measuring the angle formed between the thigh and the leg (Fig. 105).

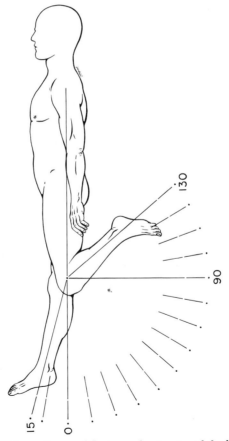

Figure 105. Range of flexion and extension of the knee.

The knee is then flexed passively by the examiner or actively by the patient, and the angle between the thigh and the leg is measured. Normally, this angle of flexion ranges from 135 to 150 degrees (Fig. 105). A simple, useful but less precise way of comparing flexion of both knees is by comparing the distance between the heel and the buttock when each or both knees are flexed as far as possible. Flexion contractures (limitation of extension) of the knee often complicate chronic involvement of this joint. Varying degrees of subluxation or dislocation of the knee are most often the result of posterior displacement of the tibia on the femur, or occasionally from destruction of one condyle and supporting plate of the tibia. When, as a result of such destruction, the tibia is dislocated laterally or medially, abnormal lateral or medial mobility is present even though the range of flexion and extension of the knee is limited.

Sometimes a catch or jerky motion can be felt or seen during passive flexion and extension of the knee when the joint space harbors loose bodies. On repetition of the motion the catch tends to occur at the same position on the arc of movement. The knee may lock or become fixed suddenly in partial extension while flexion from the point of limitation may remain relatively unrestricted.

Stability

Two basic maneuvers will usually supply information concerning stability or ligamentous relaxation of the knee.

Collateral Ligaments. Instability of the knee involves the collateral ligaments more frequently than the cruciate ligaments. The stability of the collateral ligaments may be evaluated in the following manner: With the patient's knee in complete extension the examiner fixes the femur with his left hand while he grasps the ankle with his right hand and attempts to adduct and abduct the leg on the femur in a rocking fashion. Normally, there is practically no motion; increased mobility indicates relaxation or tear of the medial or lateral collateral ligament. A loss of articular surface from a destructive process in the joint also may contribute to any instability revealed by this maneuver. If pain is elicited by this maneuver, it may indicate a lesion of a collateral ligament or a meniscus as described under palpation (see p. 163).

The knee should be observed for evidence of deformity and instability while the patient is standing. Weight bearing on an unstable knee may disclose a considerable degree of genu valgum (knock knees) or genu varum (bowlegs) which may not be readily apparent from the manual maneuver described or when the knee does not bear weight.

Cruciate Ligaments. Instability of these ligaments may be detected as follows: The patient is examined in a sitting position with the knee flexed to 90 degrees. The femur is held in a fixed position, preferably by the patient's hands, while the examiner attempts alternately to pull and push the tibia forward and backward. Normally there is only little or sometimes no excursion of the leg on the femur. Abnormally increased forward excursion of the tibia on the femur indicates instability of the anterior cruciate ligament, whereas increased posterior mobility and excursion point to instability of the posterior cruciate ligament. When abnormal excursion of the leg on the femur is present during this maneuver, it is known as a positive "drawer sign." Confirmation of. anteroposterior instability thus demonstrated may be obtained by repeating the maneuver with the leg and thigh extended. Any anteroposterior movement in this position is abnormal.

Muscle Strength

Evaluation of the strength of the quadriceps femoris or other muscles of the thigh and leg may be difficult in the presence of contractures or a painful knee. A simple method for grading muscle strength with particular reference to the quadriceps femoris is as follows: Complete inability to contract a muscle is graded as "absent" muscle strength. Muscle strength is considered "poor" when the patient is able to move his leg with some support but cannot raise the leg against gravity; "fair" when the leg can be extended against gravity through the full range of motion permitted by the joint, but the leg cannot be extended through the full range of motion when additional resistance is applied; and "good" when the muscle is somewhat weakened and not normal but still can function against some resistance applied to the leg in addition to gravity. Muscle strength is considered "normal" when the patient is able to extend his leg against considerable resistance applied to the leg.

If the patient when sitting or supine can raise the leg and foot against gravity, the strength of the quadriceps may be evaluated further by the application of variable amounts of resistance to the act of extension. Early degrees of atrophy of this muscle may be detected by palpation over the medial aspect of the quadriceps (vastus medialis) while the patient actively raises the extended leg against gravity. Functional weakness of the quadriceps can be observed when the patient attempts to rise from a low chair (height less than 17 inches) or from a squatting to a standing position without the use of his hands or other supports. Function of the gastrocnemius and soleus muscles can be evaluated by noting whether or not the patient can walk on his toes with his heels off the ground. Function of the hamstring muscles may be evaluated by having the patient attempt to flex his leg against force exerted by the examiner; frequently this test can be performed most easily with the patient prone.

Suggested Reading for Additional Information

1. Moseley, H. F.: Textbook of Surgery. Ed. 3, St. Louis, C. V. Mosby Company, 1959, pp. 1162–1178.
2. Hollinshead, W. H.: Anatomy for Surgeons. New York, Paul B. Hoeber, Inc., 1958, vol. 3, pp. 772–796.
3. DePalma, A. F.: Diseases of the Knee. Philadelphia, J. B. Lippincott Company, 1954, 840 pp.
4. Lewin, Philip: The Knee and Related Structures: Deformities, Diseases, Disabilities. Philadelphia, Lea & Febiger, 1952, 914 pp.
5. Turek, S. L.: Orthopaedics: Principles and Their Application. Philadelphia, J. B. Lippincott Company, 1959, pp. 637–695.

CHAPTER TWELVE

THE ANKLE AND FOOT

ESSENTIAL ANATOMY

The Ankle Joint

The ankle (talocrural) joint is a true hinge joint whose movement is limited almost entirely to plantar flexion and dorsiflexion. It is formed

169

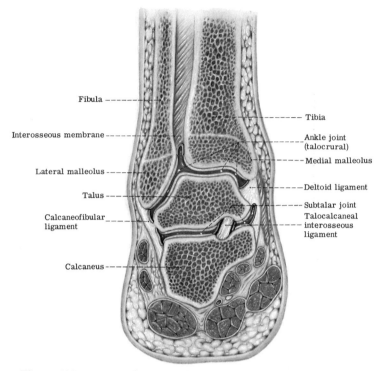

Fibula

Interosseous membrane

Lateral malleolus

Talus

Calcaneofibular ligament

Calcaneus

Tibia

Ankle joint (talocrural)

Medial malleolus

Deltoid ligament

Subtalar joint

Talocalcaneal interosseous ligament

Figure 106.   Frontal section through the ankle (talocrural) and subtalar joints. The distribution of the synovial membrane is indicated by the blue coloring.

by the distal ends of the tibia and fibula and the proximal aspect of the body of the talus. The tibia forms the weight-bearing portion of the ankle joint whereas the fibula gives lateral stability beyond the articular surface of the tibia and forms the mortise of the ankle joint. The fibula articulates on the side of the tibia and does not bear weight. The tibial and fibular malleoli extend downward beyond the roof or tibial portion of the joint and envelop the talus in a mortiselike fashion that gives lateral stability to the joint. The medial malleolus of the tibia projects inferiorly to articulate with the medial surface of the trochlea tali, and the lateral malleolus of the fibula projects inferiorly to articulate with the lateral surface of the trochlea tali (Fig. 106).

Articular Capsule, Synovial Membrane, and Ligaments of the Ankle

The articular capsule is lax and weak on the anterior and posterior aspects of the ankle joint but is tightly bound down by special ligaments on both sides (Fig. 107). Anteriorly in the midline the capsule extends from the tibia to a point approximately 1 cm. distally on the neck

170

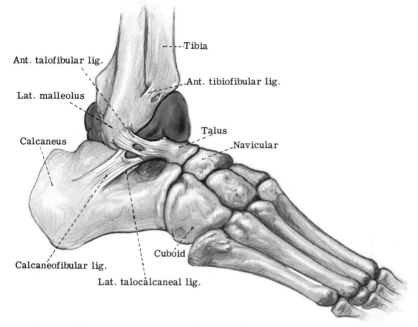

Ant. talofibular lig.

Lat. malleolus

Calcaneus

Tibia

Ant. tibiofibular lig.

Talus

Navicular

Cuboid

Calcaneofibular lig.

Lat. talocalcaneal lig.

Figure 107.   Lateral aspect of right ankle (talocrural) articulation showing the distribution of synovial membrane when distended.

of the talus. The articular capsule is less extensive posteriorly than anteriorly. The inner surface of the capsule is lined by synovial membrane. The synovial articular cavity of the ankle joint usually does not communicate with any other joints, bursae, or tendon sheaths in the region of the foot or ankle.

The ankle has strong medial and lateral ligaments, which contribute to the lateral stability of the joint. The medial or deltoid ligament is the only ligament on the medial side of the ankle. It is a strong, triangular-shaped, fibrous band that tends to resist eversion of the foot and may be torn in eversion sprains of the ankle. The lateral ligaments of the ankle consist of three distinct bands forming the posterior talofibular, the calcaneofibular, and the anterior talofibular ligaments. These ligaments may be torn in inversion sprains of the ankle.

Tendons, Tendon Sheaths, and Retinacula Adjacent to the Ankle

All the tendons crossing the ankle joint lie superficial to the articular capsule and are enclosed for part of their course in synovial sheaths, which usually are about 8 cm. long. On the anterior aspect of the ankle the extensor tendons (tibialis anterior, extensor digitorum longus, extensor hallucis longus) and their synovial tendon sheaths overlie the

171

articular capsule and synovial membrane. The tendons and tendon sheaths of the tibialis posterior, flexor digitorum longus, and flexor hallucis longus are located on the medial side of the ankle posteriorly and inferiorly to the medial malleolus; all three of these muscle tendons are plantar flexors and supinators of the foot. The tendon of the flexor hallucis longus is located more posteriorly than the other flexor tendons mentioned; it lies beneath the Achilles tendon for part of its course. The common tendon of the gastrocnemius and soleus (the Achilles tendon) lies superficial to the tendon of the flexor hallucis longus and is inserted into the posterior surface of the calcaneus where it is subject to external trauma, various inflammatory reactions and to irritation from bony spurs beneath it (Fig. 108). The Achilles tendon is separated from deeper structures by a pad of adipose tissue. On the lateral aspect of the ankle, posterior and inferior to the lateral malleolus, a synovial sheath encloses the tendons of the peronei longus and brevis; these muscle tendons extend the ankle on the leg (plantar flexion) and evert the foot. Each of the tendons or groups of tendons adjacent to the ankle may be involved separately in traumatic or disease processes.

Thickened fibrous bands hold down the tendons that cross the ankle in their passage to the foot. There are three sets of these fibrous bands or retinacula. The extensor retinaculum consists of a superior

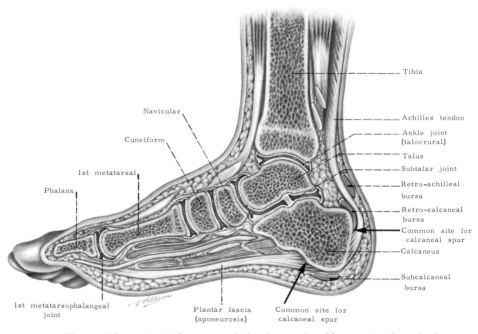

Figure 108. Sagittal section of the foot and ankle passing through the great toe. Common locations of bursae in the region of the heel are shown in blue and common sites for calcaneal spurs are shown by arrows.

part (transverse crural ligament) in the anterior and inferior portions of the leg and an inferior part (cruciate ligament) on the proximal portion of the dorsum of the foot. The flexor retinaculum (laciniate ligament) is a thickened fibrous band on the medial side of the ankle. The peroneal retinacula form two fibrous bands, a superior one and an inferior one, which bind down the tendons of the peronei longus and brevis as they cross the lateral side of the ankle.

Intertarsal and Subtalar Joints and the Foot

The intertarsal joints provide additional mobility to the foot since motion in the ankle is almost entirely limited to plantar flexion and dorsiflexion. The intertarsal joints allow the foot to be inverted and adducted (supinated) or everted and abducted (pronated). Since the foot is arched, the weight of the body is transmitted anteriorly to the heads of the metatarsals and posteriorly to the calcaneus; the latter structures are the weight-bearing portions of the foot in contact with the ground. If the arch of the foot is to be adequately preserved during the strain of weight bearing, the intertarsal joints must be firmly braced; consequently, the plantar surface of the foot is supported by unusually strong intertarsal ligaments which bind the tarsal bones together and prevent the arch of the foot from collapsing. The arch of the foot and the tarsal bones are supported also by the plantar aponeurosis, the short muscles of the foot, and long tendons which cross the ankle in their passage into the sole of the foot.

Subtalar Joint. The subtalar (subastragalar) joint is a particularly important intertarsal joint since it permits inversion and eversion of the foot. Sometimes the term, "subtalar joint," is used to refer to the talocalcaneal joint or the posterior articulation between the talus and the calcaneus. However, the subtalar joint, as the term is used clinically, is a functional unit which includes not only the posterior talocalcaneal joint but also the talocalcaneal portion of the talo-calcaneo-navicular joint and the talocalcaneal interosseous ligament which lies between these joints. The articular capsule and synovial membrane of this joint are tightly·bound to the bones composing the joint and allow little if any distention of the articular cavity. The "subtalar joint" describes the total articulation between the talus and the calcaneus and is responsible for most of the motions of inversion and eversion of the foot (Figs. 106 and 107).

The relative lengths of the first and second metatarsal bones are variable. Ordinarily the first and second metatarsals are about the same length or the second metatarsal is shorter than the first. However, in some individuals the second metatarsal may be longer than the first. Shortness of the first metatarsal bone tends to be hereditary and is usually present in the atavistic type of foot. A short or unstable first metatarsal bone tends to place additional strain on the second metatarsal and adjacent structures in the mid-tarsal area and to subject the second metatarsal and mid-portion of the foot to added trauma. This may be of significance in predisposing the foot to disorders of the longitudinal arch and fore part of the foot and also may make the second and third metatarsals susceptible to injury such as march fractures.

The plantar aponeurosis or fascia is a fibrous structure of great strength which extends from the calcaneus forward as a relatively narrow band and then divides about the middle of the foot into portions for each of the five toes. The plantar aponeurosis becomes thinner as it extends distally in a fashion similar to that of the palmar aponeurosis in the hand and fingers. The area of the plantar aponeurosis near the attachment of the plantar fascia to the calcaneus is particularly subject to the effects of trauma, inflammatory reactions, and bony spur formation (Fig. 108).

Metatarsophalangeal and Interphalangeal Joints

The anatomy of the metatarsophalangeal joints and the proximal and distal interphalangeal joints of the foot closely resembles the anatomy of the corresponding joints in the hand (see "Essential Anatomy" in Chapter 8). Each of these joints has an articular capsule lined with synovial membrane. The extensor tendon completes the capsule dorsally, the collateral ligaments strengthen the capsule on its sides, and plantar ligaments support the plantar portion of the capsule. The metatarsophalangeal joints normally undergo little flexion, and the articular capsules and synovial membranes are tighter than they are over the corresponding metacarpophalangeal joints in the hand.

Bursae

The largest bursae in the foot are commonly located over the first and fifth metatarsophalangeal joints and about the heel. The bursae about the heel are likely to occur in three locations: (1) between the skin and the Achilles tendon, (2) between the Achilles tendon and the posterior aspect of the calcaneus, and (3) between the skin on the sole of the foot and the plantar surface of the calcaneus at the attachment of the plantar fascia (Fig. 108). Subcutaneous bursae are likely to develop in areas which are subject to most of the abnormal weight bearing or friction. Thus a bursal reaction may form between the thickened skin (callus) and the underlying bony prominence of the first metatarsal head in a hallux valgus deformity of the great toe or under the callus over the prominence of a proximal interphalangeal joint in a hammer toe deformity.

INSPECTION

The foot and the ankle are observed while the patient is standing, walking, and in a nonweight-bearing position. Both feet and ankles are compared anteriorly, posteriorly, and from the sides for evidence of swelling and atrophy, deformities of the foot and toes, location of calluses, and bursal reactions, subcutaneous nodules, cutaneous changes, edema, and appearance of the nails (Figs. 109 through 115). It is helpful to note the location of calluses and bursal reactions in the foot, since their presence indicates areas of abnormal pressure or friction as described. In deformed feet, calluses and bursal reactions may occur in unusual positions, corresponding to the location of pressure points.

Swelling in Joints of Foot and Ankle and Adjacent Structures

Effusion or synovial swelling involving the ankle (talocrural) joint is most likely to cause swelling or fullness over the anterior aspect of the joint since the distribution of the synovial membranes is more extensive in this area (Figs. 107 and 114). Mild swelling of this joint may not be apparent on inspection but can often be detected by careful palpation. Posterior swelling of the ankle joint in the depression between the malleoli and the Achilles tendon may be difficult to localize to the ankle joint because of other structures in this area which may be involved separately or pushed out by an underlying synovitis of the ankle joint. Thus it is necessary to differentiate the superficial, linear swelling localized to the distribution of tendon sheaths from the more diffuse fullness and swelling due to involvement of the ankle joint. Synovitis of the intertarsal joints may occasionally cause an erythematous puffiness or fullness over the dorsum of the foot. Inflammation of ligaments which hold the fore part of the foot together may result in weakening and stretching of the supporting ligamentous structures. When this occurs, the metatarsals spread, and the width of the fore part of the foot is increased. Metatarsal spread thus occurs in some patients with rheumatoid arthritis and often is associated with the more conspicuous findings of hallux valgus and synovitis of the metatarsophalangeal joints. A resulting increase in thickness of the fore part of the foot may keep all or some of the toes from touching the floor when the patient is sitting with the feet in a resting position.

Abnormal Positions of the Foot

Inspection of the foot may reveal lowering of the longitudinal arch (pes valgoplanus or flatfoot) or abnormal elevation of the longi-

175

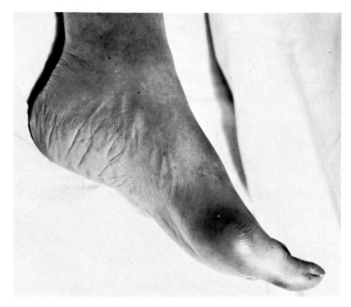

Figure 109.   Acute gouty arthritis with maximal reaction over the medial aspect of the first metatarsophalangeal joint. The involved area extends well beyond the joint proper and exhibits all the manifestations of acute inflammation: swelling, red discoloration, heat and exquisite tenderness. (Reprinted from Hench, P. S.: Gout and Gouty Arthritis. In Cecil, R. L.: A Textbook of Medicine. Ed. 7, Philadelphia, W. B. Saunders Company, 1947, p. 676, Fig. 85.)

tudinal arch (pes cavus). Talipes equinus is the position of the foot in plantar flexion and often results from contracture of the Achilles tendon with elevation of the heel and depression of the fore part of the foot (Fig. 115). This tends to occur in bedridden patients. The presence of varus or valgus of the heel is determined by noting deviation of the foot to either side of an imaginary vertical line dropped along the longitudinal axis of the lower extremity. Normally, if this vertical line is dropped from the middle of the patella, it should fall between the first and second toes. Inversion of the foot (supination) exists when the sole of the foot is turned inward, and eversion of the foot (pronation) exists when the sole of the foot is turned outward. Adduction of the foot is present when the fore part of the foot is displaced inward in relation to the midline of the leg. Abduction of the foot occurs when the fore part of the foot is displaced outward in relation to the midline of the limb. The positions of adduction and inversion (varus) or abduction and eversion (valgus) are often combined in deformities of the foot. These abnormalities of the ankles and feet may be associated with abnormalities of the knee such as genu varum (bowlegs) or genu valgum (knock knees).

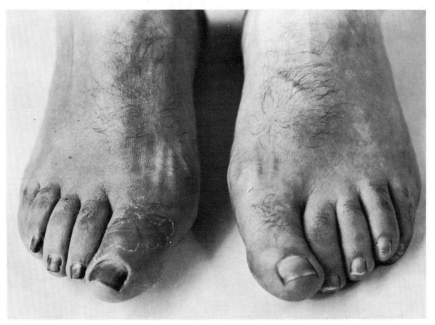

Figure 110. Subsiding attack of acute gouty arthritis in the right first distal interphalangeal joint. The skin over the affected area is peeling.

Abnormal Gaits Associated with Deformities of the Foot

Toe-Out Gait. A toe-out gait associated with an outward displacement of the fore part of the foot in relation to the midline of the leg may develop in patients with abnormalities of the foot and ankle. Patients with painful ankles or feet may splint movement of the foot and ankle by lateral deviation of the foot. This enables the patient to walk by rolling the foot from the lateral to the medial side; this replaces the normal heel-and-toe rolling gait and avoids painful motion in the ankle and joints of the foot. This lateral deviation of the foot often results in an eversion deformity, with the talus and navicular bones being displaced medially and downward and dropping of the longitudinal arch so that the patient tends to walk on the inner aspect of his foot. Thus the foot assumes a flat position, and if there is arthritic involvement of the intertarsal joints, the foot may become stiff and rigid. With the foot rotated externally, walking tends to result in increased pressure over the first metatarsophalangeal joint with weight rolling off the side of the big toe in such a manner as to push the big toe further into a more severe hallux valgus deformity. The eversion and lateral deviation of the foot tend to exert additional strain on the medial ligaments of the knee and thus may force the knees into

177

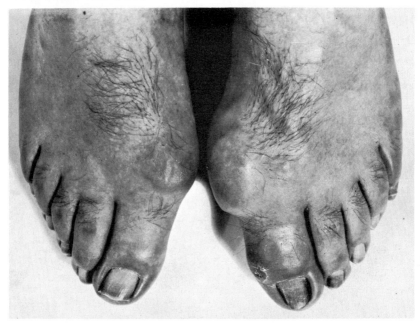

Figure 111.   Large tophus over region of the left first metatarsophalangeal joint in a patient with chronic tophaceous gout.

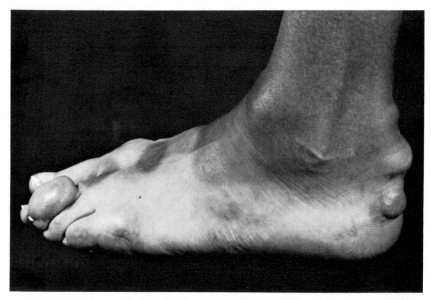

Figure 112.   Tophi over the region of the Achilles tendon and in the third toe due to chronic tophaceous gout.

178

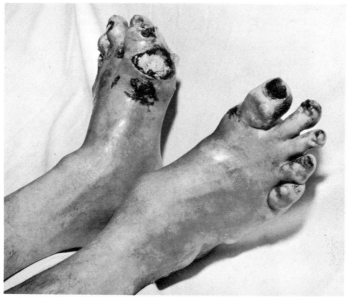

Figure 113. Advanced tophaceous gout with ulcerations of skin overlying deposits of urate and areas of necrosis.

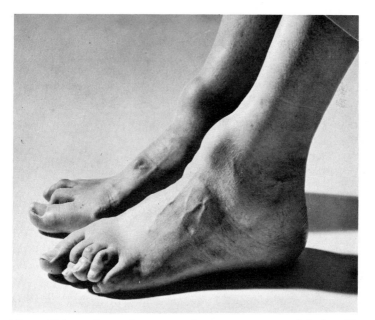

Figure 114. Synovial cysts on the anterior aspect of both ankles in a patient with rheumatoid arthritis. The cyst in each ankle communicates with the joint cavity and represents a visible distention of the synovial membrane of the joint. Hammer-toe deformities in both feet are also present and the toes do not touch the floor surface because of the deformity and the swelling of the affected metatarsophalangeal joints.

179

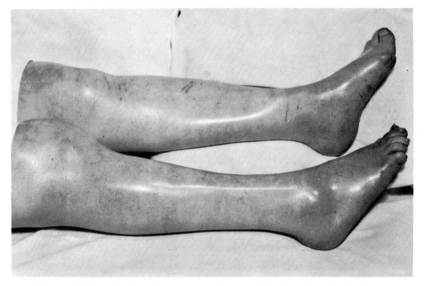

Figure 115.   Bilateral equinus position of the feet in a bedridden patient with rheumatoid arthritis. Contractures of the Achilles tendons have elevated the heels and caused plantar flexion of the feet. Prolonged disuse has also resulted in shiny and atrophic skin of the legs.

a genu valgum (knock-knee) position. The toe-out gait is awkward and fatiguing. The abnormalities just described are commonly found in feet affected by rheumatoid arthritis but also may occur in persons without evidence of this disease.

Toe-In Gait.   The toe-in or pigeon-toed gait is the result of an inward displacement of the fore part of the foot in relation to the midline of the lower extremity and is often congenital in origin. This deformity increases weight bearing on the outer side of the foot, lessening pressure on the first metatarsophalangeal joint. The inward deviation of the fore part of the foot in this condition is often associated with inversion of the foot (supination).

Abnormal Conditions of the Toes

Hallux Valgus.   The most common deformity of the great toe is hallux valgus (Fig. 116). Hallux valgus is a lateral or outward deviation of the great toe resulting in an abnormal angulation and rotation at the first metatarsophalangeal joint. The first metatarsal bone deviates medially, increases the width of the fore part of the foot and produces a prominence of the first metatarsal head. A callus and bursal reaction are commonly found over this prominence on the medial aspect of the great toe at the metatarsophalangeal joint. If the hallux valgus deformity of the great toe is marked, the big toe may overlap or underlie the second toe.

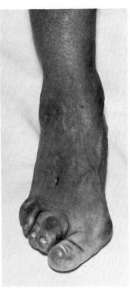

Figure 116.   Hallux valgus deformity of great toe with spread of the fore part of the foot and a bursal reaction over the medial aspect of the first metatarsophalangeal joint. Hammer-toe deformities with corns are present in the second, third, fourth, and fifth toes.

Limitation of motion at the first metatarsophalangeal joint is called "hallux rigidus."

Hammer Toes, Cockup Toes and Other Deformities of Toes. The typical hammer-toe deformity consists of hyperextension at the metatarsophalangeal joint, flexion at the proximal interphalangeal joint, and extension of the distal interphalangeal joint that produce a clawlike appearance (Figs. 114 and 116). However, in some instances the distal interphalangeal joint remains straight, and the tip of the toe touches the floor; this condition is sometimes referred to as "mallet toe." A callus or corn often develops over the prominence of the proximal interphalangeal joint. The second toe is the digit most often involved in a hammer-toe deformity and frequently is associated with a hallux valgus deformity of the big toe.

A cockup deformity of the toe consists of dorsal displacement of the proximal phalanx on the metatarsal head which becomes depressed toward the sole of the foot where it can be readily palpated. This deformity causes the tip of the toe to be elevated above the surface on which the foot is resting (Fig. 117). A cockup toe represents subluxation of the metatarsophalangeal joint and is associated with arthritic involvement of the metatarsophalangeal joint, whereas the more common hammer toe may occur with or without arthritic involvement of the foot.

There also may be lateral displacement of the proximal phalanx on the metatarsal head in any of the toes like that in the big toe with a hallux valgus deformity. This lateral deviation of the toes occurs in a manner similar to ulnar deviation of the fingers in the hand and sometimes results in overlapping of the toes on each other.

181

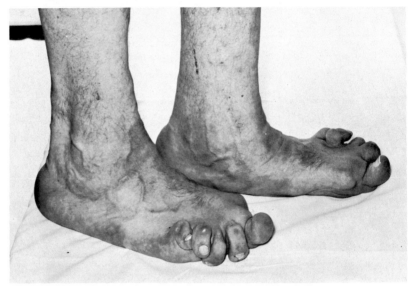

Figure 117.   Cockup deformities of the toes due to subluxation of the metatarsophalangeal joints in the fourth and fifth toes of each foot. The longitudinal arch is flat in both feet and there is eversion (pronation) of the left foot caused by abnormality of the subtalar joint. This patient has rheumatoid arthritis with involvement and resulting deformities of the other metatarsophalangeal joints.

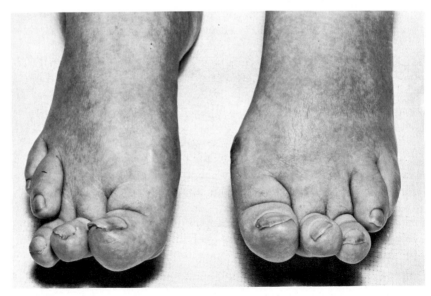

Figure 118.   Severe hyperextension deformities associated with subluxation of the interphalangeal joints in the first, second, and third toes of each foot due to rheumatoid arthritis, resulting in flail toes.

182

Hammer toes, and cockup-toe deformities or various combinations of the two often are the result of articular damage and inflammatory changes in the articular capsule and surrounding ligaments of the meta-tarsophalangeal joints of the second, third, fourth and fifth toes. Severe articular damage of the interphalangeal joints of the toes may produce hyperextension deformities of the phalanges of the toes (Fig. 118).

PALPATION

The Ankle Joint

With the patient seated or supine, the patient's right foot is sup-ported by the examiner's right hand while the fingers of the examiner's left hand palpate the soft tissues overlying the anterior aspect of the joint (Figs. 119 and 120). The right hand grasps the heel snugly and compresses the area behind and beneath the medial malleolus with the palm and thenar muscles, while the fingers of the same hand apply firm pressure behind and beneath the lateral malleolus in order to distend the articular capsule and synovial membrane anteriorly where they can be palpated more easily with the examiner's other hand if synovitis is present in the ankle. Then the fingers or thumb of the examiner's left hand may palpate lightly over the depressed area of the joint space

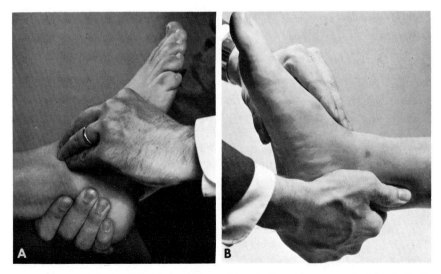

Figure 119. Palpation of the ankle. *A.* Lateral aspect of right foot. *B.* Medial aspect of right foot. The patient's foot is supported by the examiner's right hand. With this hand the examiner firmly compresses the posterior aspect of the articular capsule and synovial membrane in order to distend the articular capsule and synovial membrane anteriorly where they can be palpated by the fingers of the examiner's left hand if synovitis is present (see text for details).

183

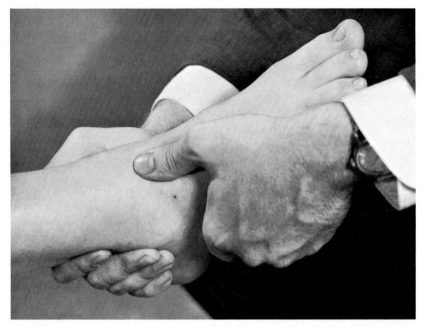

Figure 120.   Palpation of the ankle when the examiner uses his thumb instead of his fingers. The patient's foot is supported with one hand as described for Figure 119 while the thumb of the examiner's other hand palpates over the anterior aspect of the joint to detect tenderness and soft-tissue swelling in this area.

on the anterior aspect of the joint to detect abnormal fullness or soft-tissue swelling in this area. If synovial swelling or effusion of the ankle joint is present, it is most likely to be palpable anteriorly since the reflection of the synovial membrane is more extensive over the anterior aspect of the joint than elsewhere (Fig. 107). It may be difficult to outline the margins of a distended synovial membrane with certainty in this area due to the presence of overlying structures. Care should be taken to avoid stretching the skin and soft tissues on the anterior aspect of the ankle with the hand which is positioned posteriorly since the resulting tightness of the skin may make deep palpation and the detection of synovitis more difficult or impossible. The anterior aspect of the ankle may be examined also by using both thumbs as shown in Figure 121.

Warmth and tenderness may be increased over the ankle joint, but if they are due to synovitis in this area, they should be localized to the involved region.

The Heel

A painful heel may be caused by an osseous spur or spurs, inflammation in the Achilles tendon, a calcaneal bursa, or a calcaneal fat pad.

184

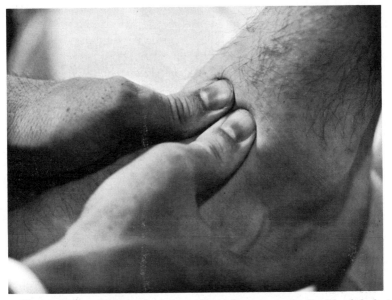

Figure 121.   Palpation of the ankle (alternate method). The left foot is supported by the fingers of both hands. Both thumbs are used to palpate firmly (note blanched nails) over the anterior aspect of the ankle joint.

Painful heels also may be caused by fractures, osteomyelitis, periostitis, bone tumors, or strain on the attachment of the plantar fascia or other trauma to ligaments and soft tissues about the heels. Careful localization of swelling and tenderness by palpation may help reveal abnormalities in any of these structures.

The Achilles tendon is subject to localized inflammatory reactions and trauma. Palpable swelling and tenderness on the back of the heel may result from inflammation of superficial structures such as a subcutaneous bursa or from inflammation of deeper structures such as the bursa which lies between the calcaneus and the Achilles tendon just proximal to the point of its attachment (Fig. 108). It may be difficult to distinguish the more superficial swelling about the tendon from the deeper bursal reaction. However, differentiation of these sites of involvement by palpation is important when possible since the deeper bursal reaction often signifies inflammation due to a systemic disease such as rheumatoid arthritis or ankylosing (rheumatoid) spondylitis, whereas the more superficial swelling of an injured tendon or a subcutaneous bursa is often caused by trauma or excessive friction from a tight shoe. An inflamed bursa in the region of the Achilles tendon is often associated with thickness of the skin overlying the bursa, forming a callus. Xanthomatous, tophaceous, fibrous or rheumatoid nodules may be palpable in the affected part of the tendon.

185

Pain on the sole of the foot near the heel may be due to inflamma-tion or trauma at the site of bursae or the attachment of the plantar fascia to the calcaneus (Fig. 108). Localized tenderness to palpation over the anterior and plantar aspects of the bony prominence of the calcaneus may result from a bursal reaction located between the cal-caneus and the skin. Usually the bursal reaction is near the attachment of the plantar fascia to the calcaneus. It may overlie a bony spur which sometimes develops on the calcaneus in this area.

As noted previously, a painful heel may be associated with a bony spur on the calcaneus. The two most common sites for spurs in the heel are: (1) the plantar surface of the calcaneus near the site of attachment of the plantar fascia and (2) the insertion of the Achilles tendon in the posterior aspect of the calcaneus (Fig. 108). The pain associated with calcaneal spurs is due primarily to the inflammatory reaction in adjacent soft tissues rather than to the bony spur itself. Calcaneal spurs are often asymptomatic and are best detected in a lateral roentgenogram of the foot.

Intertarsal Joints

The intertarsal joints are palpated distal to the ankle between the examiner's thumbs on the dorsum of the foot and his fingers on the plantar surface of the foot. Swelling, tenderness, and warmth are the main physical findings which may be detected by palpation. Usually these signs are present on the dorsal rather than the plantar aspect of the foot. Although tenderness may be localized, swelling is rarely local-ized to any particular intertarsal joint (except occasionally the talo-calcaneo-navicular joint) and usually is detected as generalized thicken-ing or fullness over the dorsum of the foot. Swelling in this region must be differentiated from localized tenosynovitis of the extensors of the foot.

Metatarsophalangeal Joints

The metatarsophalangeal joints are palpated between the exami-ner's thumb and forefinger as shown in Figure 122. The thumb is placed on the dorsum of the foot, and the fingers of the same hand are posi-tioned on the plantar aspect about 0.5 cm. proximal to the position of the thumb in order to locate the metatarsal heads (Fig. 122).

The examiner palpates the metatarsal heads on both the dorsal and plantar aspects of the foot but especially through the soft tissues over the plantar surface. The soft tissues on the plantar aspect consist of thick skin, superficial fascia and adipose tissue. The fascia and adipose tissue serve as a padding between the bones and skin, in addition to the underlying articular capsule and the synovial membrane of the meta-

186

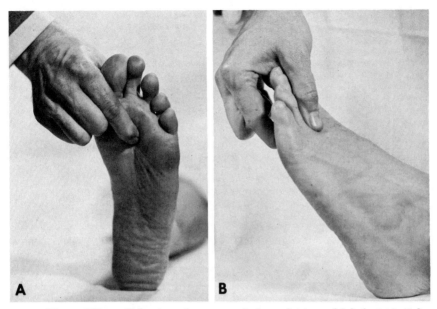

Figure 122.   Palpation of metatarsophalangeal joints of left foot. *A.* Volar view. *B.* Lateral view. The forefinger is palpating deeply between the second and third metatarsal heads. Note how far proximally the metatarsal heads actually are located. See text for details.

tarsophalangeal joints. The soft-tissue thickness varies with the amount of synovitis and with the thickness or atrophy of the fat pads and other subcutaneous tissues. Palpation over the metatarsal heads not only gives information about the soft-tissue reactions in this area but also may reveal deformities or subluxation in the metatarsophalangeal joints. Subluxation of a metatarsophalangeal joint produces a dorsal displacement of the proximal phalanx on the metatarsal head, and the metatarsal head becomes more than usually prominent on the plantar aspect of the foot where it can be palpated easily. Subluxation of a metatarsophalangeal joint commonly produces a cockup deformity of the toe as described in the paragraphs on "Inspection" (see p. 181).

In the presence of chronic synovitis (for example, rheumatoid arthritis) involving the metatarsophalangeal joints and supporting ligaments, there is a loss of the normal fat pad under the metatarsal bones, and spreading of the metatarsals is likely. When the soft-tissue reaction and swelling subside, the metatarsal heads lie directly under the skin where they are readily palpable and are also subject to additional trauma.

Palpation for synovitis of the metatarsophalangeal joints is performed by starting proximally between the shafts of any two adjacent metatarsal bones. As the thumb and fingers of the examiner are gradually moved distally toward the metatarsophalangeal joint, the area between the metatarsal bones is palpated. Normally, the palpating finger can extend a short distance into the groove between adjacent metatarsal bones and the groove between adjacent metatarsal heads. However, the second and third metatarsal bones are tightly bound together in the normal individual so that it is normally difficult to palpate between them satisfactorily. The region over the metatarsal head and the groove between adjacent metatarsal heads are firmly palpated for evidence of synovial thickening or distention by rolling the examining forefinger over and between the plantar surfaces of the metatarsal heads (Fig. 122). Normally the synovial membrane cannot be palpated in the groove between adjacent metatarsal heads, but in the presence of boggy synovial thickening or distention, this groove may be partially obliterated by the abnormal distribution or reaction of the synovial membrane. The soft-tissue swelling of a distended synovial membrane also may be palpated over the plantar surface of the metatarsal head, partially obscuring the bony prominence of the metatarsal head. Palpable swelling and tenderness between any two adjacent metatarsophalangeal joints may represent a local inflammatory process accompanying a neuroma or may represent synovial swelling in the metatarsophalangeal joint. The soft-tissue swelling of synovitis is palpable on both sides of the involved joint.

Tenderness to palpation over the metatarsophalangeal joint is particularly helpful in detecting abnormal involvement of this joint and is often present when there is synovitis in the joint, but local heat or redness is usually absent. Tenderness of the metatarsophalangeal joints can be evaluated by firmly palpating each joint between the thumb and the forefinger (Fig. 122) and also (but with less localization) by grasping the fore part of the patient's foot with one hand and squeezing the metatarsal heads together between the thumb on one side of the foot and the fingers on the other side.

Interphalangeal Joints

The proximal and distal interphalangeal joints of the toes are palpated in a manner similar to palpation of the corresponding joints in the fingers. The examiner's thumb and forefinger are used to palpate the medial and lateral aspect of the joint (Fig. 123). Synovitis in the interphalangeal joints is usually detected best on the medial and lateral aspects of the joint while varying degrees of pressure are applied by the palpating fingers to determine the presence of swelling, tenderness or warmth.

Other Abnormalities of the Foot and Ankle

Tenosynovitis Near the Ankle. The tendons crossing the region of the ankle are enclosed for part of their course in synovial sheaths as described on page 171. When these synovial tendon sheaths become

188

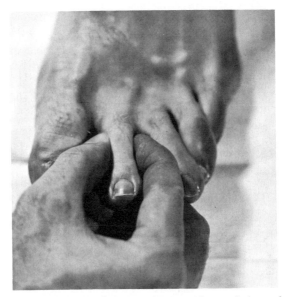

Figure 123. Palpation of the left second proximal interphalangeal joint of the toe. The examiner's thumb and forefinger are used to palpate the medial and lateral aspects of the joint to detect swelling and tenderness.

inflamed (tenosynovitis), it is important to differentiate the superficial linear swelling and tenderness of tenosynovitis from the more diffuse swelling and fullness of synovitis in the underlying ankle joint. The swelling and tenderness of tenosynovitis can be localized by palpation over the distribution of the tendon sheaths and is linear in nature, whereas the swelling and tenderness of synovitis in the ankle joint when it is palpated anteriorly is found in the distribution of the synovial membrane over the anterior aspect of the joint. A tenosynovial reaction may occur in the extensor tendon sheaths over the anterior aspect of the ankle. Sometimes a tenosynovial reaction may result in linear tenderness and swelling below and behind the medial or lateral malleoli. The sheath of the posterior tibial tendon which is located on the medial aspect of the ankle is particularly subject to tenosynovitis. Tenosynovitis frequently causes pain on movement of the involved tendon. Thus, inversion or eversion of the foot against resistance may cause pain when there is a tenosynovial reaction on the respective medial or lateral aspect of the foot or ankle, and extension of the foot against resistance may be painful when there is a tenosynovial reaction of the extensor tendons on the anterior portion of the ankle. However, failure to produce pain with these maneuvers does not exclude a tenosynovial reaction.

Morton's Toe (Metatarsalgia). Morton's toe or metatarsalgia is characterized by severe crampy or burning pain in the anterior portion of the foot, often under the fourth metatarsal head, which usually

189

occurs with weight bearing while wearing shoes. The pain is often relieved by sitting down and removing the shoe. It is usually unilateral and is more common in females than in males. This condition is often associated with a neuroma of the plantar digital nerve, which is usually located between the third and fourth toes. Firm palpation may reveal tenderness over the third interspace and sometimes a palpable tumor there. There also may be hypesthesia on the lateral aspect of the third toe and the medial aspect of the fourth toe.

March Foot.   The march foot is caused by severe or prolonged use of the foot, such as strenuous marching, and usually results in a transverse fracture of the metatarsal shaft. The second metatarsal is affected most frequently and the third metatarsal next most frequently, but any of the metatarsals can be involved. Localized pain develops over the dorsum of the fore part of the foot, causing the patient to limp. The most common and significant finding on physical examination is palpable tenderness and swelling over the fracture. The diagnosis is confirmed by roentgenographic examination of the foot.

MOVEMENT AND RANGE OF MOTION

Movement at the ankle (talocrural) joint is limited almost entirely to plantar flexion and dorsiflexion. From the normal position of rest in which there is an angle of 90 degrees between the leg and foot (labeled 0 degree on Figure 124), the ankle joint normally allows about 20 degrees of dorsiflexion and about 45 degrees of plantar flexion (Fig. 124).

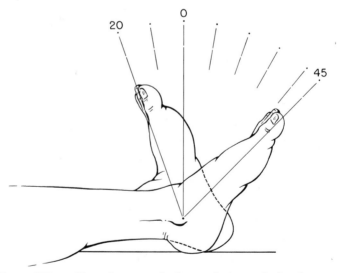

Figure 124.   Normal range of plantar flexion and dorsiflexion in ankle joint.

190

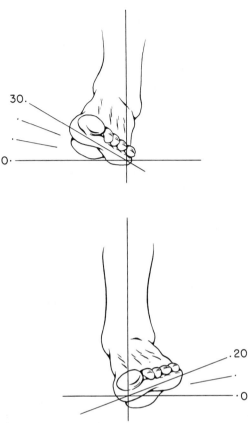

Figure 125.   Normal range of inversion (supination) and eversion (pronation) in subtalar joint.

Inversion and eversion of the foot occur mainly at the subtalar (subastragalar) articulation. Inversion of the foot (supination) exists when the sole of the foot is turned inward and eversion of the foot (pronation) exists when the sole of the foot is turned outward. From the normal position of rest, the subtalar joint normally permits about 20 degrees of eversion and about 30 degrees of inversion (Fig. 125).

Muscle weakness and stretching of inflamed ligaments in the midportion of the foot and in the region of the intertarsal joints may be associated with characteristic deformities and limitation of motion in the foot. A condition known as pes planovalgus is said to be the most common midtarsal deformity in patients with rheumatoid arthritis.

The metatarsophalangeal joint of the great toe flexes about 80 degrees and extends about 35 degrees (Fig. 126). The metatarsophalangeal joints of the second to fifth toes move only about 40 degrees in either flexion or extension. The proximal interphalangeal joints

191

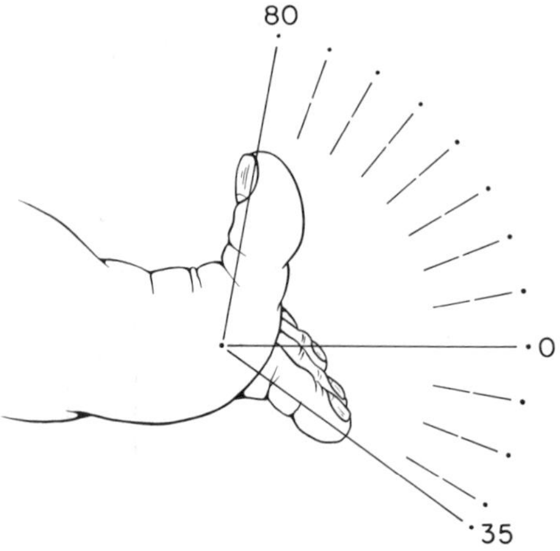

80

Figure 126. Normal range of extension in the first metatarsophalangeal joint and normal range of flexion in second to fifth metatarsophalangeal joints.

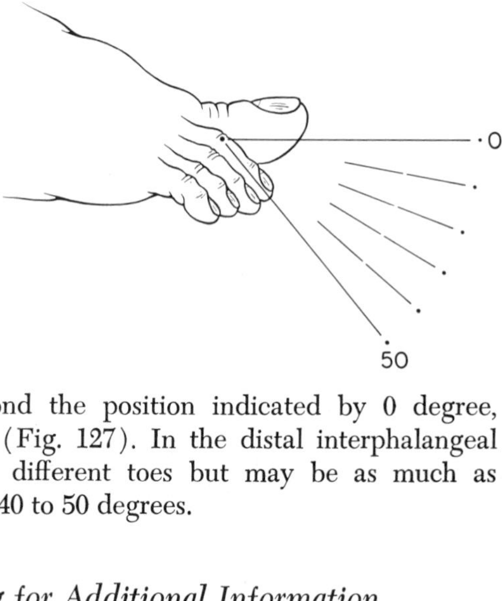

•O

•35

Figure 127. Normal range of flexion in proximal interphalangeal joint of toe. This joint does not extend beyond 0 degree.

•O

50

normally do not extend beyond the position indicated by 0 degree, but do flex about 50 degrees (Fig. 127). In the distal interphalangeal joints extension varies in the different toes but may be as much as 30 degrees and flexion is about 40 to 50 degrees.

Suggested Reading for Additional Information

1. Lewin, Philip: The Foot and Ankle: Their Injuries, Diseases, Deformities and Disabilities. Ed. 4, Philadelphia, Lea & Febiger, 1959, 612 pp.
2. DuVries, H. L.: Surgery of the Foot. St. Louis, C. V. Mosby Company, 1959, 494 pp.
3. Hollinshead, W. H.: Anatomy for Surgeons. New York, Paul B. Hoeber, Inc., 1958, vol. 3, pp. 831–882.
4. Lake, N. C.: The Foot. Ed. 4, Baltimore, Williams & Wilkins Company, 1952, 466 pp.
5. Hauser, E. D. W.: Diseases of the Foot. Ed. 2, Philadelphia, W. B. Saunders Company, 1950, 415 pp.
6. Calabro, J. J.: A Critical Evaluation of the Diagnostic Features of the Feet in Rheumatoid Arthritis. Arth. & Rheumat. 5:19–29 (Feb.) 1962.
7. Kuhns, J. G., and Potter, T. A.: Painful Feet. In Hollander, J. L.: Arthritis and Allied Conditions: A Textbook of Rheumatology. Ed. 6, Philadelphia, Lea & Febiger, 1960, pp. 1131–1161.

INDEX

References to illustrations are in italic type.

194